TO DO NO HARM

A Journey Through Medical School

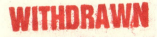

TO DO NO HARM

A *Journey Through* *Medical School*

PHILIP REILLY, M.D., J.D.

 Auburn House Publishing Company
Dover, Massachusetts

Library of Congress Cataloging in Publication Data

Reilly, Philip, 1947–
   To do no harm.
   1. Reilly, Philip, 1947–   2. Physicians—United
States—Biography.   3. Medical students—United
States—Biography.   4. Medical education—United
States—Philosophy.   5. Yale University. School of Medicine.   I. Title.
[DNLM: 1. Education, Medical—personal narratives.   2. Students,
Medical—personal narratives. W 18 R362t]
R154.R355A3   1987   610'.7'1173   [B]   86-26576 ISBN
0-86569-162-2

To My Wife, Nancy, and
To My Son, Thomas Marshall

FOREWORD

You, the reader, are about to embark on a guided tour of Yale Medical School led by a medical student, with four years compressed into several evenings of intense, emotionally laden reading. It is a tale you will not forget. If you are a health professional, the stories and sketches will jar many personal memories of your own previous journey through student training. If you are a premedical student you will find the experience both threatening and demystifying. If you are a health care consumer you will gain new insights into the psyches of the doctors and nurses who care for you. If you are sentimental about the honorable medical profession and the trust you accord your physician you will have some rude awakenings and will, perhaps, lose some of your unquestioned adoration. If you are jaded about the imperfections and selfishness of the members of this learned profession you will gain insight into the typical foibles that all of us possess.

Dr. Philip Reilly, your tour guide, has written a diary of the experiences in medical school that have molded him into the doctor he is today. He has successfully refrained from retrospective editing of the notes he recorded during his four-year journey. He has chosen to write about those events which had the greatest impact on him while he was a student in training.

By describing his experiences, Dr. Reilly shares a number of practical and ethical issues with the reader: Is it deception to call a medical student a doctor? Should all available means to treat a patient or save a patient's life be carried out when the patient is protesting—either "rationally" or "irrationally"? When is it time to let a patient die? What thoughts race through the mind of a medical student when performing the first rectal exam, bone marrow biopsy, or spinal tap? Are most patients discharged from the hospital because they no longer need acute care or because their insurance has been depleted?

The author has written extensively about his own personal struggle to understand pain and suffering, sickness and recovery, dying and death. He has confronted his feelings honestly and with refreshing candor. He describes the tension between his teachers' admonition to study and treat patients with scientific objectivity and his own emotional, subjective involvements with the patients who were assigned to him for diagnostic and treatment plans to be presented to his demanding, sometimes unforgiving, instructors. He describes his confrontation with the issue of truth-telling to patients—what to tell, how much to tell, when to break devastating news. Coming to medical school with a background of legal training and experience and with deep respect for individual autonomy and self-determination, he learned during his medical training why physicians since the days of Hippocrates have been devoted to the concept of the best interests of the patient, which is easily (and often accurately) perceived outside the profession as paternalism. He jumped through the hoops required of all students on their way to a medical degree, but not without stumbling and balking many times, as all students do, trying to maintain his own sense of self while developing maturity.

Philip Reilly's story is engagingly told, filled with impressions and rich with similes and analogies. One can almost see, hear, smell, and feel the patients he describes. Often they resemble people we have known well—not stereotypes, but individuals. Because the diary was contemporaneously recorded, one can see a bumbling, scared, wet-behind-the-ears medical student gradually transformed and "professionalized" into a competent, self-assured young doctor. Although this story is personally unique, it touches upon the stories of all medical students.

I feel particularly fortunate that Philip has shared his experiences with me by writing this book. I knew him for seven years before he entered medical school and have followed his career development through residency training, board certification in internal medicine, and his present successful practice as Medical Director at the Eunice Kennedy Shriver Center for Mental Retardation in Boston. His perspectives may be somewhat atypical, reflecting more maturity at times than that of residents who were "teaching" him, but for the most part he played by the team's rules, despite personal misgivings.

Philip Reilly will always be an inquiring student. His medical school experiences were an important step in his development as a compassionate and caring physician. His book is worth reading.

Margery W. Shaw, M.D., J.D.

2 November 1986
Houston, Texas

PREFACE

During the fall of 1976, 40,569 students filled out 371,545 applications to become members of the next freshman class in 119 medical schools in the United States. After countless committee meetings, one hundred thousand "personal" interviews, and millions of dollars spent by the applicants on long-distance phone calls, air fare, and cheap hotels, the medical schools mailed out 25,714 acceptances to fill 15,493 seats. A total of 5186 persons received at least two offers, and 565 individuals got bids from at least five schools. The 1976 record belongs to a talented, but somewhat insecure, applicant who received a high of 16 acceptances (and 30 rejections).

When the dust had settled and final students had found their seats, the class of 1981 included 11,549 men and 3944 women. It was the first time in history that female matriculants had exceeded 25 percent of the total. The average freshman was twenty-three years old. Slightly more than 1000 freshmen were at least twenty-eight years old, and the oldest accepted male and female students were both forty-two. A total of 6513 (16.1 percent) minority-group students had been in the applicant pool. This included 3299 members of the four minority groups (black American, American Indian, Mexican American, and mainland Puerto Rican) targeted for greater representation in U.S. medical schools.

A total of 2954 people applied for one of the 102 places in the freshman class at Yale Medical School. When the music finally stopped, seventy-four men and twenty-eight women were sitting in Yale chairs. I was one of them.

I had heard that Yale traditionally landed extraordinarily talented students. In fact academic standards were not helpful in sorting them out. Just about everybody had done remarkably well at a highly prestigious college. One-half of my classmates had graduated from Harvard, Yale, or Stanford. Many had published their first scientific papers and had career plans to which they had already pledged the next decade of their lives. Some of the older students had completed advanced studies in other fields (genetics, French literature, engineering) but wanted to study medicine badly enough to be willing to start over. Others had led even less conventional lives. In the first days came the first rumors. He had spent a year on a religious trek through India. She was a mathematical wizard who had made it big as a professional gambler. That guy had lived on a beach in Tahiti for a year; this woman had been lead singer in a rock group for the last decade. As the months passed we would discover that, even discounting exaggerations, we were in fact a very talented group.

We would also learn and relearn another fact: Prior accomplishments did not count. Even the most brilliant student would still have to confront the mountains of memorization in anatomy and spend long hours with a wrinkled cadaver. Everybody would have to study those immensely thick books, spend ungodly hours on the hospital wards, and adapt to a state of perpetual ignorance.

This book focuses mainly on the *clinical* education that I received in medical school. I do not devote much attention to "book" courses (biochemistry, pharmacology, genetics). Although these are the scientific foundations upon which medical science rests, the learning process here is not dissimilar from undergraduate education. I have emphasized how we learned to examine and care for sick people. The choice of words here is crucial; we did not learn from healthy persons. Our teachers were the sick, the dying, and even the dead. They helped us to become doctors. This education changes people. It makes the world view of the doctor unique.

Innumerable books have been written about the years a young doctor spends as an intern or resident. But despite the incredible intensity of the years a doctor spends as a house officer, I believe that his or her attitudes about respect for persons, about what constitutes sickness and health, and about fears of death and dying, to name a few, are well formed before that first patient is ever admitted. I wanted to watch these attitudes take shape in myself; that is the story I have to tell.

I began to write this book a few days before I started my freshman year at Yale Medical School. My goal was simple. I wanted to record as faithfully as possible the experiences of becoming a doctor. I wished neither to dramatize those four years nor trivialize them. I harbored no illusions that my experiences could be used to construct some ultimately accurate description of medical school. I did not fancy myself an amateur sociologist, nor was I driven to reform medical education. I simply wanted to compile an honest record about what I thought was one of the most unique "passages" in our society.

The crucial task was to study myself and, to a lesser extent, my teachers, my patients, and my fellow students. Becoming a doctor is an emotional steeplechase, loaded with obstacles that trip one many times before the finish line. It is an intense, fast-paced race, and if you are one of the runners, there is little time to reflect on it. For four years I doggedly stuck to my plan. Nearly every day I tried to review my experiences, to ask others how they felt about our training, and to record my thoughts before they slipped away.

I was troubled by two problems. How could I deliver the most accurate report of my impressions? I wanted the reader to stand in my shoes, to see what I saw, to smell what I smelled, to hear what I heard. I decided that it was crucial to keep my impressions fresh. For four years a pocket-sized recorder, not much bigger than a deck of cards, perched on my desk next to my medical textbooks, crying out for equal time (which it rarely got). Once in a while I even carried it with me to class or the hospital. But I felt wrong doing this, and I never recorded anybody's voice without his or her consent. I did scribble down comments made by doctors, nurses, patients, or fellow students, for they often captured a thought better than had I.

The second, much more troubling, problem focused on the issue of privacy. Because my comments were spontaneous and unedited, they would reveal a lot about myself as well as about the world I had entered. I wanted to be open, so I tried to resist the urge to edit. Nevertheless, I had to confront the fact that the persons whose lives I brushed during my medical education might be opposed to my decision to tell this story. Out of respect for them, I have changed all the names and embellished or altered many anecdotes to protect the privacy of others.

Hindsight is a tough editor. Looking back, what I wrote occasionally seems naive and sometimes seems foolish. But it was important that I try to capture how a student becomes a physician. Perhaps a few insights will counter the inevitable foibles.

This book is a memoir of my education at the Yale University School of Medicine. The professors, the house officers, and my fellow students taught me a great deal, and my first patients taught me even more.

I wish to acknowledge and thank Patricia Cook, who cheerfully typed this manuscript and offered several helpful comments.

CONTENTS

A little panic fear grew in his mind. As his imagination went forward to a fight, he saw hideous possibilities. He contemplated the lurking menaces of the future, and failed in an effort to see himself standing stoutly in the midst of them. He recalled his visions of broken-bladed glory, but in the shadow of the impending tumult he suspected them to be impossible pictures.

FROM THE RED BADGE OF COURAGE
BY STEPHEN CRANE

Chapter 1

ANATOMY

Breathless from three flights of stairs and months of antici-
pation, I stopped before the heavy glass doors that isolated
this wing from the rest of the old brick building. The
September sun fired three shafts of sharply angled light,
each marking a doorway that opened on the dim corridor
beyond. A simple block-lettered sign crudely taped at eye
level confirmed the address: "Section of Human Anatomy—Restricted Area." Meant to ward off the curious, this
sign seductively beckoned newcomers like me. In the
dissecting rooms off this corridor, I would spend the better
part of the first year of my medical education pursuing the
mysteries of the human body. The voyage to this world had
been long, and although classes did not begin for three
days, I had to explore it now.

The corridor doors yielded silently. An air current
slapped me with a sickly sweet pungency—the odor of a
disinfectant mixed with dime store perfume. Just inside on
the right was a giant x-ray viewing box, a huge sheet of
white plastic that overlay a panel of fluorescent lights.
Some careful soul had neatly arranged a dozen smoothly
dark x-ray films in three rows. Beneath each hung a tiny
white card with a typed explanation. I flipped the toggle
switch, the light flickered and held, and twelve human

1

heads materialized. I remembered Janus, the two-faced household god whose busts had graced the foyers of wealthy Romans.

The little card below the first film solemnly informed me that its image was of a child with hydrocephalus. In the center of the brain was a great, dark, gracefully curving shape, a sea gull's shadow cast upon sand. According to the card, increased fluid pressure had greatly dilated the cerebral ventricles. What, I wondered, were cerebral ventricles? Next to the hydrocephalic head was the film of an *internal carotid artery angiogram*. A great vessel rose majestically through the neck, took several sharp bends, and broke into a mass of rivulets that ran, patternless, in all directions. "How many branches of the internal carotid can you identify?" sneered the little card. "None," I admitted, retreating hastily.

Glass display cases lined the left side of the corridor. A gruesome collection of Nature's mad sculptures floated eerily in giant bottles. These were the creatures that crawled the landscapes of nightmares. The first deformed baby was called *sirenomelus*. Through the ancient amber fluid I could see the head and torso of a child, but there were no legs or feet. Instead the body tapered, like the tail of a reptile, to a point. Had the birth of such a baby on a Greek island thousands of years ago spawned tales of mermaids?

The next case housed three infants who had died at birth with *craniorachischisis*. It looked as though they had been murdered with an axe. A great fissure started at the top of the head and ran the length of the back. The brain and spinal column had herniated outside the body. One of the babies faced forward. His skull was horribly flattened, and his eyes bulged froglike to dominate the face. His ears were set very low, and his head sunk deeply into his chest; there was no neck. He shamed Hollywood's most bizarre celluloid monsters. In the center of the shelf below was a bottle proclaimed by its display card to be "extremely rare, at least seventy-five years old." A normal-looking baby floated in a three-foot-high jar. His umbilical cord ran upward to a rounded structure into which a square window had been cut. Through it one could see that the placenta still clung with white gossamer threads to the wall of the uterus. The label explained that after the death of a pregnant woman, the uterus *and* the baby had been removed at autopsy. This explained the great rarity. Today, women rarely die in labor, and the baby certainly could be saved.

One case of curios stretched into the next. At the far end of the hall stood a magnificent collection of Neanderthal skulls. But, what I really wished to see lay behind the doors to a room marked C–359. According to a diagram on the bulletin board, three as yet unknown classmates and I would spend our mornings dissecting the cadaver on table 21.

The door to C–359 was ajar. The room was shaped like a shoe box; seven narrow stainless steel tables stood in a neat row along its length. Seven cadavers lay waiting. Curiously colored, orange-red, rubber blankets shrouded the bodies. A giant gray lamp, the shape of an inverted kettledrum, hung over each table. I stepped forward and lit the nearest lamp. A cone of light brightened a circle of red rubber. These lamps would guide us into the secret nooks and crannies. Hesitant and frightened, I cautiously circled the tables.

Except for its unusual inhabitants, the room was simple enough. Four deep steel sinks jutted from one wall. Thick bars of yellow soap lined the narrow ledge above them. Next to the sinks stood a huge, scarred wooden cabinet. Inside on simple plywood shelves were scattered an odd collection of saws and drills. What ghastly chores would I perform with these? At the end of one shelf lay four hinged wooden boxes, about the size of hat boxes. I gingerly opened one. A human skull grinned back. The box seemed to shut itself! In one corner of the ceiling hung a single television console. Beneath it and just to the left stood a full human skeleton. Tiny springs and wires had replaced tendons and ligaments. It was small, about five feet. I shuddered. Someone had told me that many of these skeletons were the remains of beggars from Bangladesh. After starving to death, their bodies were dipped in acid, picked clean in "insect tanks," and shipped by some enterprising businessperson to the United States. Their bones earned more in death than they had in life.

I held my breath and tiptoed to my table. I grasped one corner of the surprisingly heavy blanket and slowly pulled back until I could see flesh. A layer of thick, clear plastic lay underneath the outer shroud. Through it I could see what vaguely resembled a human leg. The shape was right, but the color was all wrong. In death I expected a pasty white, like the underbelly of a fish, but this was much worse. The skin was a ghastly gray-brown; ugly black hairs bristled against the plastic sheet. A wave of revulsion swept over me; this was worse than the bottle babies! I dropped the blanket, backpedaled to the door, and retreated. Perhaps it was better to let my curiosity simmer for a few more days; the official start of "Gross Anatomy" was soon enough.

The class of 1981 assembled for its first lecture at 8:30 on the morning of September 12 in the anatomy lecture room. Low-ceilinged, darkly shaded, and overheated, it was an unpleasant place. Fifteen rows of tightly linked, battered oaken seats receded from a green chalkboard. It was a wedge of space that induced claustrophobia. More than one hundred twenty people crammed the hall. Nearly everyone clutched a knapsack, shopping bag, or satchel, in which was stuffed a change of clothes, a lab coat, and a small collection of instruments. The luggage-laden crowd mimicked a bus station in Providence or Albany. This was only a stopping place; the real destination was upstairs.

Looking about, I concluded that like me most people had bartered lab coats from the second-year students, a group that seemed ominously eager to sell everything that reminded them of anatomy. One shop had a virtual monopoly on the sale of medical supplies in New Haven, so it determined what the well-dressed medical student would wear. The anatomy smock (which I had purchased from a neighbor for five dollars) was a battleship gray, short-sleeved, collarless wrap-around. Over the weekend, sales of used dissecting kits had also been brisk. I had acquired two scalpels, a pair of latex gloves, a scissors, a plastic ruler, two forceps, and four probes—all for the princely sum of three dollars. My wooden-handled probes looked as though they had been passed through several generations.

As a tall, white-haired, white-coated gentleman entered the front door, the class quickly quieted. His name was Dr. Thomas Frost, and he had been teaching anatomy at Yale for nearly forty years. He had shared the first day of medical school with several thousand students, and he knew that our confident faces masked more than a few terrors. Twice that summer I had dreamed cadaver dreams—dark, vague stories of corpses come to life. I had heard the usual anecdotes: A few medical students vomited on their first day in the dissection room, some people were unable to eat meat for weeks, and (rarely) the cadaver even ended a fledgling doctor's career. How would I react?

For the first few minutes Dr. Frost took a businesslike approach, reading the simple rules of conduct and cleanup to be followed during and after the day's dissection. Attention to these housekeeping chores calmed me a bit. That done, he paused, fumbled for a bit of paper in his pocket, and gazed about the room. He would retire in June, so this was the last time that he would shepherd students into the study of gross anatomy. He waited patiently until the last whisper had died, and then he spoke.

"It is quite natural to be afraid on the first day," he said gently. "I was. We all fear death and the unknown. But I promise you that your fears will melt away as your eagerness to pursue the body's mystery grows. Let me help you by reading the advice of Leonardo da Vinci, one of the great anatomists. He wrote, 'O Speculator, concerning this machine of ours, let it not distress you that you import knowledge of it through another's death, but rejoice that our Creator has ordained the intellect to such excellence of perception.'" Seemingly caught up in the words, Dr. Frost paused ever so slightly. After that he returned to his businesslike manner. "OK. Let's go upstairs and begin to work."

Rather than let ourselves be randomly assigned to a team, Paul and Kathy, two people whom I had met at registration, and I had agreed to work together. They had found a fourth, a woman named Nancy, whom I met as we filtered through the milling crowd to our table. For a moment we just stood dumbly, clutching our dissecting kits, laboratory notebooks and atlases, eyeing the red rubber blanket that covered our cadaver. Breaking the spell, Paul, a tall bearded man in his late twenties, walked to the other end of the table and began to remove and fold the blanket. Kathy tugged the single clear sheet of plastic that had been beneath the rubber shroud and quickly stowed it. We confronted our cadaver.

A large man lay face up on the narrow steel table. His head, hands, and feet were wrapped in wet, bulky gauze. His legs were strong and athletic looking, but he had obviously enjoyed a good meal. His chest and belly formed a small mountain. I silently groaned. The only consistent advice that I had heard over the summer was to scramble for a table with an emaciated cadaver. "If you get an obese one," I had been warned, "you spend the first two weeks shoveling fat, and you won't learn any anatomy until October."

As we surveyed his massive torso, Nancy read from the "cadaver list." Our man had died two summers ago at seventy-eight from congestive heart failure. That was all we would ever know about him—his age and the diagnosis listed on his death certificate. A fantasy floated through me: This bon vivant who relished Viennese pastry had played a little joke on death. Two years after his heart had stopped, he had emerged from his briny barrel to captivate four medical students for six months. I wanted desperately to know more about him. What kind of work had he done? Perhaps he had been a physician. Did he have children and grandchildren? How had they reacted to his decision to donate his body to a medical school? Why had he decided to do so? He had probably lived in Connecticut. Had he rooted for the tragic Red Sox or the hated Yankees? Most of all, I wanted to know his name. I was not examining a cadaver; I was looking at a dead man, the first dead man I had ever touched. He deserved to have a name. I wondered what my new lab partners would think if I suggested one. Glancing down at his thick, sleek torso, I remembered an old detective show that I had occasionally watched, a show full of dead bodies. What the hell!

"Our friend needs a name, don't you think?" I suggested somewhat sheepishly.

I was greeted with three quizzical smiles, but no outright guffaws or rejections.

"Let's call him Kojak!" I urged. "He reminds me of Telly Savalas."

Kathy looked gravely at our man, his face still wrapped

in gauze, and then grinned. "Kojak it is," she agreed. There was no dissent. In death he had a new name.

According to our dissecting manual (a 100-page guide to the lab work), our first job was to "reflect the skin and fascia [What, I wondered, is fascia?] from the anterior body wall." To do this we had to make three giant incisions, forming the shape of a capital *I*. The vertical line would run from "the jugular notch to the pubic symphysis" (right down the middle of the chest and belly), and the horizontal lines would stretch from shoulder to shoulder and from hip to hip. The idea was to create two giant flaps that could be reflected to each side, exposing the chest and belly muscles. Nancy claimed the right to make the first incision. After arguing with us a bit about what exactly represented the midline, she put her small blade to the base of his neck and began to draw a long incision southward. The skin, leathery from two years in a tub of salty water, resisted her attack, and soon all four of us were cutting on dotted lines that we had drawn with magic markers to guide our wobbly hands.

Working quarters were tight. I leaned over Kojak's thighs and plunged my scalpel through the tough skin just below the belly button. I drew the blade firmly toward the black pubic hair. As the skin split, tightly packed globules of butter-yellow fat, a vast storehouse of unused energy, emerged. In a few minutes we had connected our various incisions, and we were ready for the second step in our dissection. "Remove all the fat between the skin and the anterior body wall," the manual commanded.

By now we were all wondering about the same question. "How deep do you think that this fat goes?" asked Paul.

"Let's find out," said Kathy, as she rummaged through her meager instrument kit.

Kathy and Paul retracted the skin of his belly in opposite

directions, and I sliced a deep furrow into the yellow mound: one inch, two inches, three, about four inches deep.

"We'll be here all day just removing fat," groaned Nancy.

"I have this awful feeling that you are right," Kathy commiserated.

The students to our right had been blessed with a frail, old female who could not have weighed ninety pounds. I noticed that they were nearly finished scraping away the mere quarter inch of fat that their lady had carried to death. Below one skin flap we could already see the "anterior layer of the rectus sheath," which housed the rectus muscle (the one that hurts when you do sit-ups). We had to get moving!

"Let's pair off and each take a side," urged Kathy, as she glanced at the wall clock.

Paul and I took Kojak's right. The task was conceptually simple. First we had to separate the skin from the fat, then we had to separate the fat from the muscle that it covered. But, it was tricky to clean the skin flap without making "button holes," tiny rents that occurred when one scraped too vigorously or when the knife slipped. In a few minutes we had developed a strategy. Starting at the corner where the hip line intersected the center line, we cautiously flayed fat from the underside of the skin until we had cleared a few square inches. It was like a maddening effort to peel an uncanceled postage stamp from an envelope. But once we had a good corner, we could bend the skin back and harvest some fat.

Stuffed into tight latex gloves, my hands were hot and uncomfortable. The fat globules melted as we scraped them from the skin, and my grip grew slippery. Abandoning the final barrier between me and the cadaver, I stripped my gloves off and tossed them into the metal waste pail at the foot of the table. It was time to get dirty.

As it liquified, the fat felt greasy and revolting. Bits of

dead flesh quickly worked themselves under my nails. I suppressed a silent wave of nausea. Almost involuntarily, I lifted my left hand to my nose. My fingers reeked of phenol and camphor and wintergreen. I looked at my hand. The nails were sparkling clean, as though I had just finished washing a huge load of dinner dishes. This was the work of the phenol, a powerful organic solvent. It was an odor that would linger faintly on my fingertips, no matter how much I scrubbed, for the next six months.

We cut the fat into small cubes as though we were serving birthday cake. It gave way easily to the new blades, and in seconds we had removed several slabs.

"Now what do we do?" questioned Paul, gesticulating at the growing mound of fat that was perched precariously on the table edge.

"It's hard to think about it in these terms," I replied, "but I guess that this guy's fat is now trash." We dropped the slabs into the steel bucket.

The morning sped past. By noon our trash can was overflowing with paper towels and human fat. Nevertheless, we had failed to complete the day's simple dissection assignment: to "locate the deltoid branch of the thoracoacromial artery," a vessel that branches to supply blood to the pectoralis, the big muscle beneath the nipple. After a brief discussion, we agreed that we could catch up tomorrow and decided to quit for the day. We neatly replaced the sheet and rubber blanket, cleaned our instruments, scrubbed our hands long and hard in the deep sinks, and strolled out chattering happily.

I never got sick, but it was difficult that first day, as I unwrapped my tuna fish sandwich, to believe that my hands were really clean.

Anatomy quickly became the cynosure of my life. Week after week from quarter past eight until noon the class

had tightened and contracted the fingers. It took several hours and a half-dozen scalpel blades to flay the leathery skin from each finger without cutting the tendons we sought to understand. Working between stiffened fingers, we were forced to remove the skin in tiny slivers. Twice I nicked myself when the knife slipped. This was bad, but not nearly as bad as nicking one's partner, an embarrassment that I barely avoided. We worked steadily until our own fingers ached, but we were rewarded. Late in the afternoon we were able to tug on the various extensors and flexors in the forearm, and watch the fingers dance. Even in death the hand obeyed the laws of Newtonian mechanics! We had created a macabre marionette.

As one month dissolved into the next, the task of dissection acquired a certain routine. To dismember a body now seemed no more unnatural than to collect tolls on a highway or process bank loans. There was, however, an experience that pranced strangely in our future. One morning we would unwrap the white shroud that hid Kojak's face from our eyes and hands and knives. Would that be another test? Would we be able to cut into his eyes? Saw through his skull? Remove his brain? Would he become more human (more difficult to dismember) once we confronted his face?

It happened in mid-January. The manual instructed us to study the "muscles of expression and arteries of the face." The first command was to "remove the gauze that has protected the face." The four of us gathered at the head of the table, drawn in a tight circle, as though we wished to exclude everyone else from this intimate event. Kathy lifted the heavy head off its wooden pillow, and Paul unwound the endless yards of wet gauze.

His hair was auburn—not a fleck of gray in his seventy-eighth year. How could that be, I wondered? Perhaps the chemicals in which Kojak had floated for two years had dyed his hair? He had bushy brown eyebrows and long lashes. His nose was large, bumpy, and coarsely chiseled.

Had he broken it playing football in high school? His mouth was open, his jaw fixed. I counted six teeth. Kathy beamed a penlight into his mouth and discovered that one molar was solid gold! During the autumn we had occasionally wondered about Kojak's looks. Carried away by naming him, I had predicted that he would be brown-eyed, bald, and blessed with a hooked nose. I was wrong. He had green eyes, green like the sea on a cloudy August day, and he did not look like Telly Savalas.

Our first job was to locate the parotid (salivary) gland, its duct, the facial artery and vein, and the masseter muscle (the powerful chewing muscle). The parotid gland nests in front of and below the ear at the edge of the cheek. The short duct runs forward over the masseter, a finger's breadth below the bony zygomatic arch to empty into the mouth opposite the second upper molar. As we labored that morning to dissect the gland and its duct, we found ourselves trying to avoid Kojak's eyes. Finally, by common consent, we draped a towel over his forehead and nose. Somehow, it made things a lot easier.

I remembered one great fact from anatomy that day: No branches of the facial nerve emerge from the anterior side of the gland, so it can be exposed quickly by the surgeon. A few months later the fact that I knew this so impressed an ear, nose, and throat surgeon that he bought me lunch! For once anatomy paid off.

It was during my anatomy course that, thanks to Dr. Frost, I became enchanted with the history of medicine. On Thursdays at noon about fifteen of us trooped directly from the lab to a seminar room where Frost lectured informally about milestones in the history of medicine. Reading from large, meticulously printed white index cards, and frequently passing around ancient medical texts borrowed from Yale's rare book collection, he imparted to us a priceless gift. He gave us a sense of belonging to an ancient and honorable discipline.

How could one not marvel at the determination of Vesalius, the Italian scientist, who learned his anatomy by stealing the bodies of crucified criminals and dissecting them under cover of night. With no preservatives or refrigeration, Vesalius had at most a day before the stink of putrefaction became unbearable. For a short time Ambrose Paré, the battle field surgeon, was my hero. Paré saved incalculable suffering by recognizing that the application of a soothing mixture of herbs was preferable to a poultice of hot tar after the amputation of a limb that had been decimated by gunshot. Da Vinci, Harvey, and, especially, Semmelweis, who showed that simply by washing one's hands between deliveries, the physician could sharply reduce the number of women who died from puerperal fever, still hold special status in my pantheon.

Besides the stories there were the drawings and models. The school's anatomy collection included an exceedingly rare series of sagittal (vertical) sections of the human head and chest cast in plaster of paris. Some German master had created these pieces—exact copies of extraordinarily difficult and rare divisions of human cadavers—nearly a century ago. One could also study human musculature by examining life-size drawings made by Italian artists in the seventeenth century.

In keeping with tradition at Yale, there were no anatomy examinations for which we were required to sit. However, we were expected to attend four "table conferences." Each consisted of a lengthy visit with one of the several instructors who circulated from table to table during the mornings. The regular visit lasted five or ten minutes, but a table conference lasted about ninety minutes. The instructor reviewed dissection and posed various questions to test our anatomical knowledge. Although they were not intended to have this effect, the table conferences terrified many of us. We grew uneasy with the prospect of making glaring admissions of ignorance in front of a professor and our peers. The privacy of a written, machine-graded exam, success at which had brought us to medical school, seemed highly desirable.

Our first conference was with Dr. Datta, a brilliant, sweet Indian woman, who seemed completely unconcerned that none of us could answer her questions. Her knowledge of anatomy was encyclopedic and her interest in teaching so intense that she had little desire to trap us with trick questions. Dr. Thorn, a taciturn Englishman, was quite the opposite. At the second conference (in late November) he asked me to point out the lines of origin of the gluteus maximus (buttocks). Trembling with ignorance, I pointed every which way at the iliac crest (the top of the hip), until he stopped me with a snort of condescending laughter and advised me to purchase an anatomy text as soon as possible. I was mortified. Fortunately, my anatomy partners and I, devastated by our encounter with Dr. Thorn, got even. In March he conducted our final conference, on the anatomy of the face and head. This time I trembled with pleasure, as I correctly named all the branches of the external carotid artery, and Kathy correctly identified the origin and insertion of the pterygoid muscles. It was difficult for Thorn, but he grudgingly admitted that this time we had "obviously studied a bit."

Early in February it dawned on me that the anatomy course would soon end. For five months the dissecting room had been the center of my universe. After developing a little dexterity and mastering a few facts, I had greatly enjoyed it. As a child I had demonstrated neither interest nor ability in handicrafts. Anatomy dissection was the first time I had ever really been required to work with my hands. The discovery that I was not a complete klutz had real therapeutic value. I even started to fantasize about becoming a surgeon! Indeed, the high point of my time in anatomy may have been when a visiting surgeon said that my exposure of the three tiny bones of the middle ear was the best that he had seen. This was my reward for two hours of painstakingly chipping bone slivers from inside the skull.

The last day of anatomy was on March 14. Dr. Frost stopped the dissection early so that those students who wished could attend a memorial service for the cadavers. Now little more than a pile of hacked-up parts, Kojak and the others would be cremated later that week. Although long dead, these humans had greatly influenced our lives, and we found the chaplain's memorial service to be appropriate.

About twenty-five of us crowded into Chaplain Edwards's familiar office. He had been a regular visitor to the anatomy lab, and his rooms harbored the only free coffee in the medical school. The ceremony was short and simple. Edwards read a few verses from the New Testament, and then a student named Harvey, whom I had not yet met, said a prayer in Hebrew. He also quoted from the Talmud the scriptural advice that a religious law could be violated if it was necessary to save a human life. In the eyes of Judaic law our learning was permissible because it was viewed as a preparation for lifesaving activity.

After the official ceremony, Paul, Kathy, Nancy, and I returned one last time to our table. Nancy had invited us to join her in a private farewell. We stood in a circle about Kojak, savoring new memories. Over the months we had become close. One night in October Paul had invited us to dinner. From cocktails to a delicious steak dinner, we had moved on to throw a magnificent drunk, highlighted by hours of dancing to old Mo-town records. Eventually, each one of us had hosted a similar evening. After a few drinks a lot of tension, and even some tears, had spilled out to mix with the laughter. Now the four of us were meeting as anatomy partners for the last time.

As we reminisced, Kathy had a crazy whim. Pulling pliers from the tool cabinet, she deftly removed Kojak's gold tooth.

"This is our souvenir," she proclaimed. "Over the years we will rotate possession of it. If we agree to pass it on by hand every few years, then we will always stay in touch."

We solemnly agreed, and Kathy was assigned to keep the tooth. Nancy had written a poem in honor of Kojak, which she wanted to read. I drew the black window shades. Paul flicked out all the lights, save for our overhead lamp. Except for the cone of light bathing the rubber shroud, the room was dark. We stood in the shadows as Nancy read. Then we quickly said good-bye. It was in the nature of medical education with its infinity of new rotations and heavy demands on one's time that the four of us never assembled again.

Chapter 2

CLINICAL TUTORIALS

Regardless of the depth of one's interest in the subject, the study of human anatomy conveyed to most physicians a palpable sense for the rich history of that art. Much of what we did in the dissection room recapitulated innumerable hours of study by our predecessors dating to the fifteenth century. This quiet sense of the past was antipodal to the exciting sense of the future that energized us on each contact with clinical medicine. Our immersion in patient care would not occur until the summer after our second year, but from the first month of medical school a program called "clinical tutorials" beckoned us to the technological wonders of modern medicine far more powerfully than anatomy had reminded us of its origins.

Clinical tutorial was not a course; it was a preview of things to come, a promise that if we stayed on track, we too would be admitted to the mystical fellowship of the cardiac catheterization lab, the neurosurgical operating suite, or the electron microscope. It did much to alleviate the frustrations of freshmen who yearned to see patients, and it helped us to create a new self-image. With each hour that we spent with clinicians we became a bit more convinced that we could enter their world.

The clinical tutorial course was organized in a simple fashion. The class was randomly divided into groups of four

and matched to a physician who had volunteered to spend
two hours each week taking us to see patients. Because this
commitment ran from September to April, the tutors were
a highly self-selected group. They really wanted to teach.
Given that these were the first physicians with whom we
would walk the wards, they would leave an indelible mark
on our notions of what it was like to be a modern physician.

On the second Monday of my medical school career, a
note in my mailbox directed me and three classmates to
meet Dr. Ben Sanders, a pediatrician who worked in the
primary care center. It was my first walk through the old
hospital basement, a warren of narrow corridors with walls
of chipped paint. Bright stripes of yellow, red, and green
paint lined the floors, and slick new plastic signs hung
overhead. A security guard reassured me that if I followed
the red line and obeyed the signs, I would soon reach
Sanders's office. Ten minutes later, however, I found myself at an unmarked door that housed an examining room
for the orthopedic clinic. An ancient secretary, who had
probably helped hundreds of my predecessors find their
way, warned me to ignore all signs and take a series of
rights and lefts.

The next door I tried, also unmarked, was the correct
one. I saw three faces, vaguely familiar from the first week
of lectures. Ron was a sleepy-eyed, gentle-faced New
Yorker who had just graduated from MIT. Neal, a powerfully built man with a super smile, had studied at Penn.
The third, a slightly built, curly-headed guy in green
corduroys and a lumberjack shirt, James, had graduated
from Harvard a few years earlier. Dr. Sanders arrived a few
minutes later. A tall, athletic-looking man in his late thirties, he had honey colored hair flecked with gray and wore
steel-rimmed glasses that struck a studious note. In just a
few minutes I concluded that his taciturn manner masked a
good humor. My first impression proved true; fate had
forged an amicable group.

Dr. Sanders had arranged for our initial visit to be devoted to a tour of the hospital. For students who had spent most of their time thus far with cadavers, the first stop required a dramatic reorientation. We followed our leader through the radiology suite into an inner chamber. We now stood before the CAT scanner. CAT stands for "computerized axial tomography," a fancy phrase for an incredible x-ray machine that "sees" the body in three dimensions, and which in the late seventies was being hailed as an ultimate diagnostic weapon. The room was jammed with computers; through thick glass one could see the giant, doughnut-shaped scanner that recalled Flash Gordon's rocket ship. The white-coated men seemed more like physicists than physicians; there was not a stethoscope in sight. At Dr. Sanders's request, the chief radiologist paused to describe the scanner's immense resolving power, its ever-expanding diagnostic capabilities, and its cost. As he spoke we watched a computerized image of cross-sections of a man's head, the internal structures depicted in vivid hues, flash across the screen. The radiologist explained that he was looking for a tiny brain tumor that might explain the patient's complaint of intermittent dizziness and nausea.

Due to its cost, the CAT scanner was at that time the focus of the debate over how to control the spiraling cost of health care. The "planners" wanted to "regionalize" the distribution of this tool. They reasoned that if a hospital purchased a scanner, it would be compelled to use it a lot to recoup its investment. The physicians who opposed external controls argued that some patients who might be saved by easy access to a CAT scanner would die if the diagnosis was delayed by several hours. I had tended to side with the economy-minded argument, but the CAT scanner's seductive charms could not go unnoticed. It was easy to understand why every radiologist in the country would want access to this awesome machine. I could feel the full force of the technological imperative washing over me.

As you read these pages, the echoes of debate over using CAT scanners have faded. Today, in the mid-eighties, the planners are debating whether to regionalize access to MRI (magnetic resonance imaging), an even more awesome and more expensive piece of diagnostic equipment. In just five years the CAT scanner has been forced to abdicate its technological throne. Doubtless, five years from now MRI will also have been replaced, perhaps by PET (positron emission tomography) scanning, a technology that allows a machine to assess the metabolic activity of various regions of the body.

The next stop on our tour was the cardiac catheterization lab, another high tech chamber, which earned the hospital "big bucks," as Dr. Sanders candidly put it. Through a window we watched as three cardiologists, gowned in mint green scrub suits, threaded a long, thin tube into a man's thigh and up his vessels to his heart. A television console hung above the table and a fancy looking fluoroscope stood nearby. As the doctors squirted dye into the catheter, a technician deftly positioned the "fluoro." The console came alive with pictures of a human heart, filling and emptying, filling and emptying, like some mysterious undersea creature captured by Jacques Cousteau.

The rest of the afternoon was a steeplechase of visits to other laboratories, the pediatric wards, the x-ray file room, the emergency room, and the cafeteria. Everyone we met was friendly, but we encountered a lot of curious grins. Had the words "first-year medical student" been tattooed on our cherubic faces? A big man, Sanders walked with a fast stride. Shorter, slower, and more timid, we followed like four ducklings behind their mama. No wonder people were smiling; we were being imprinted as sure as if we were Graylag geese!

Late that afternoon we met our first patient, a nine-year-

old girl with ash blond hair and an impish smile named
Bonnie. She was suffering from a mysterious disease called
juvenile rheumatoid arthritis. With slow, careful movements, Dr. Sanders showed us that Bonnie's elbows were
swollen and that the arc through which she could move her
arm was diminished. Her cheeks were puffy, which Dr.
Sanders explained was caused by one of her medicines.

As we were leaving, Bonnie's mother walked in, and Dr.
Sanders paused to introduce his "young doctors." I tensed.
Green medical students may prefer the protective cloak of
titles, but I thought the introduction was patently false. We
were not young doctors; we were first-year (first-semester,
first-week?) medical students. I wanted to disavow the
introduction, but I wished neither to embarrass nor offend
Dr. Sanders. Hoping that he would not notice, I solved my
ethical dilemma by reintroducing myself.

"Hello. My name is Philip Reilly, and I am a first-year
medical student."

Her reply baffled me. "Very nice to meet you, doctor."

So much for honesty. I let matters stand.

A few weeks later our class attended the premier session
of an occasional seminar series called "clinical correlations."
These seminars were intended to discuss recent scientific
discoveries that were especially relevant to patient care.
The first topic, technological advances in the diagnosis of
congenital cardiac defects, was presented in what I realized
all too soon was a classic example of medical education.
Although we had not the slightest knowledge of cardiac
embryology, the pediatric cardiologist peppered his rapid
presentation with mysterious terms like VSD, TGA, and
Fallot's tetralogy (each, I later learned, refers to a particular birth defect). Most of the talk was completely over our
heads and, I thought, a waste of time. But the instructors
seemed totally unconcerned. When a classmate inter-

rupted to say that he was confused, the cardiologist told
him not to worry. "In medicine," he said, "floundering is a
way of life."

The seminar was an exercise in technological seduction.
The doctors, who had brought along some of their "hard-
ware," reminded me of masterful salesmen. Only a few
minutes after starting a conventional lecture at the chalkboard, the cardiologist asked his colleague to cut the room
lights and redirected our attention to the ultrasound machine. This desk-sized instrument was a mass of dials that
enclosed a video screen. With a few turns of the knobs, he
brought up for us "real time" images of the beating heart of
a human infant. By freeze-framing the action he was able to
point out to novices the structural defect from which the
infant suffered. We were mesmerized. As he finished,
someone called out.

"How much is it? I'll buy it."

As the class chuckled, I guessed that this was exactly the
effect that the doctor had hoped to achieve.

By the end of the hour we were convinced of the virtues
of cardiac catheterization and ultrasonography, but no one
had mentioned the risks posed to the patient when a
catheter is threaded into the heart. Almost as an after-
thought, one lecturer acknowledged that during catheterization an infant is dosed with the equivalent of a year's
background radiation. Was there, I wondered, an increased risk for leukemia? How did one explain this to a
worried parent?

The class did not seem troubled by their inability to
comprehend the remarks about congenital heart defects.
Judging by my "applause meter," this had been the most
popular lecture thus far, which, given that we attended
about fifteen a week, was saying something. Many people
drifted to the front to fondle the equipment and ask more
detailed questions. As I squeezed through, I wondered
which classmates were reflecting on how these early "clini-

cal" discussions were shaping our images of physicians and our notions of illness. How important is pediatric cardiology to the nation's health? Three out of a thousand infants are born with congenital heart disease. This is significant, but it pales before the problems of child abuse, malnutrition, and lead paint poisoning. But there were no fancy scientific discoveries to help deal with these clinical problems, and no "clinical correlation" time had been set aside to discuss them.

It did not take long for me to realize how perceptive the cardiologist had been when he had admonished us that "floundering" was a way of life. On our second afternoon with Dr. Sanders we spent several hours trying to learn the rudiments of using a stethoscope. We marched from room to room, politely listening to the lungs of as many patients with abnormal breath sounds as he had been able to locate. The task seemed simple enough. First, we listened briefly to each other so we would have a baseline with which to compare our findings. But as I moved from patient to patient, placing the stethoscope exactly where I was told, the odd whispering noises all seemed pretty much alike. I was utterly confused by the way in which Dr. Sanders distinguished *rales* from *rhonchi*, and his confidence made my ignorance seem all the more appalling. By the end of the session I had begun to detect a difference between inspiration and expiration, but I would not have jumped for the opportunity to identify which was which.

Around five o'clock we put away our stethoscopes and Dr. Sanders took us to see two patients on whom he had been asked to "consult." The first was a little baby who looked to be about six months of age. As we surrounded his crib, Dr. Sanders decided to test our powers of observation.

"I want all of you to look at this baby and then tell me what you see."

There was a long pause as four of us bent over the chubby, sleeping infant. Hair, two eyes, a nose, a mouth, a body, four limbs, ten fingers, ten toes; a baby in a diaper in a crib. He or she looked normal to me. Was I missing something? One by one Dr. Sanders asked us to describe what we saw. All four answers were the same, but I could see by the look of dismay that he was shocked by our obtuseness.

"What about his skin? Does his skin look different?"

"No," I admitted.

"Put your finger on his chest."

I did, but my ignorance only deepened. I chose silence.

"Come on you guys," urged Sanders. "This kid is lemon yellow. He has big time liver disease. This is jaundice, and his bilirubin is thirty."

Suddenly, the cobwebs were blown away. He was right; this child was yellow. How could we possibly have failed to notice this? But we had.

"He looks normal to me," muttered Neal, his Chinese face lit with a grin.

"It's a good lesson for you. You can't see what you're not trained to find. The eye is the servant of the brain. Remember that," ordered Sanders.

The last patient we saw was a seventeen-year-old boy who had been in the hospital for two months with complications after surgery to replace a valve in his heart. He was not at all happy to see us. He barely spoke, and his face was granite as Dr. Sanders examined him. I asked two questions about the history of his illness, and to both he answered, "I don't know." I wondered whether this was a sign of his anger or if nobody had ever explained his curious illness to him.

"Do you think this boy understands his problems?" I asked Dr. Sanders as we strode down the corridor.

"Of course. He didn't answer because it was the easiest way to get rid of us."

I hoped that Sanders was right. I sure would not let anyone "crack" my chest without a full explanation, but a teenage boy might not have been able to comprehend the message. Perhaps that was partly why he was so angry. Did he see himself surrounded by people who never really talked to him? Is this what "informed consent" was all about?

As I hurried through the hospital corridors that afternoon I made my first observation about "style" in medicine. The stethoscope with which I had bumbled for several hours was much more than a mere diagnostic tool; it was, like jewelry or a necktie, a means of self-expression. Some people, especially medical students and interns, "wear" their stethoscopes draped around the back of the neck and shoulders. The studied nonchalance with which the wearers maintain this precarious perch conveys a cool, confident air, as though they were ready for action at a moment's notice. The senior residents prefer to let their stethoscopes dangle from their necks like ties. They pause at the patient's bedside, quickly survey the scene, and somberly listen. In their hands the stethoscope (this year's favorite model was the elegant Hewlett-Packard, known by its short tubing and glass diaphragm) elicits hidden secrets. The older docs, dressed in expensive suits and Gucci shoes, let their stethoscopes peek from the right coat pocket. Except for cardiologists, who carry rare scopes of unknown make (is there a Stradivarius of stethoscopes?), many "attendings" seemed to favor the cheapest models, the throwaways handed out by salesmen as promotional gimmicks. It was as though they carried the instruments only to confirm for the record what they can discern in a glance!

Although it also carried a "high technology" billing, our next clinical correlation was very different from the first. The topic was "the surgical repair of tracheoesophageal fistulas," a congenital malformation in which there is a connection between the wind pipe and the food pipe. If this condition is not promptly fixed, the patient will aspirate food and stomach acids into the lungs and die of pneumonia. Most of the hour was devoted to the dramatic tale of how physicians had developed the operations to repair this defect. But toward the end the surgeon digressed to contrast his approach to patients with TE fistulas to his approach to babies with meningomyelocele. This is the technical term for spina bifida, a birth defect in which part of the baby's spinal cord hangs in a sac outside the back. Despite surgery, the doctor explained, most babies with spina bifida are destined to life in a wheelchair. There is also a big risk of mental retardation due to problems with the circulation of cerebrospinal fluid, the watery substance that bathes the brain and nerve cord. The surgeon was painfully candid.

"Assuming that the babies are otherwise normal, I always repair TE fistulas. But, sometimes I advise parents of a newborn with a bad spinal lesion not to pursue surgery."

Hands flew up around the room. "What gives you the right to end a baby's life?" challenged one woman.

"Don't most babies who undergo surgery quickly have normal intellectual function?" asked another.

"Doesn't this decision belong to the parents?" demanded a third classmate.

The surgeon backpedaled, but only a bit. He admitted that many babies with spina bifida were not mentally retarded, and that parents should make the ultimate decision.

"But," he asserted, "the parents depend on me for the prognosis. If I think that the child's future is extremely bleak, it is my duty to make that picture very clear. The parents can make a meaningful decision only based on the facts that I know."

"Dr. Halsted, I am amazed at your words," said one student, his voice shaking. "You don't have a crystal ball. You can't really predict a child's future. One more thing. A lot of people would be pretty offended by your notion that it is best to let some babies die."

The class grew silent. This was the first time that anyone had assaulted one of the "masters." How would he react? Dr. Halsted looked past us, perhaps at the wall clock, perhaps wondering at our disrespect. A sad smile lightened a face that had been dark with anger. As he spoke his voice dropped to a whisper. I strained to hear him.

"In the next few years you will learn more about fear and uncertainty than you could ever dream. Uncertainty is the great secret of medicine. If we ever revealed the depths of our ignorance and self-doubt, our patients would suffer horribly. We owe it to them to lock these monsters in our deepest dungeons. It is true that deceit and denial sometimes form the foundations of our relationships with patients, but the charade is motivated by compassion. You'll see. By overemphasizing hard facts about a baby with a horrible prognosis, I may be saving a family a lifetime of agony. I believe that it is the right thing to do."

There was another long silence. Something special had happened. A teacher had revealed and students had learned more than either had intended.

As one Thursday slipped into the next, it seemed that our tutor had devised a master plan to make each clinical session more revealing than the next. Two weeks after Dr. Halsted's troubling remarks about "uncertainty" Dr. Sanders let us eavesdrop on a heated debate about whether a baby had a "surgical belly." A third-year resident, convinced that the infant was suffering from intussusception (a life-threatening bowel obstruction caused when the intestinal tube folds in upon itself), was trying to persuade his attending physician that the patient should be rushed to the operating room. The contrast was marked. The resident, his speech pressured and his hands dancing, was pacing like a big cat in a small cage. The senior physician, bearded and pipe-smoking, was quietly attentive. We watched as the surgeon reviewed the x-rays that the resident thought had clinched the diagnosis. Agreeing that the house officer's interpretation was correct, the older man still ruled against a fast trip to the operating room.

"But this kid could die from a gangrenous bowel. We have to open him up," said the resident, pleading like a lawyer before a judge.

"I think we can wait a few hours yet. Sometimes these things just resolve by themselves. Let's do a barium reduction [a nonsurgical treatment] and see if that helps," suggested the senior man.

"It's too risky. We should cut." The house officer was apoplectic. Only the ironclad rules of hierarchy held him back. Dr. Sanders motioned us to leave. As we walked away, I hazarded an opinion.

"That surgeon is awfully calm."

"Maybe the resident is just awfully excited," countered James.

"Being too certain or too excited doesn't help you be a good surgeon," ruled Dr. Sanders. "Don't worry, the attending will get that baby in the OR in time. He is obeying one of surgery's first rules: Don't do an emergency operation unless it is indicated. Doctors have to control their powerful need to act."

Dr. Sanders was extremely popular with the pediatric residents. Naturally, he was besieged with hallway consultations as he walked the wards with us. A few minutes after leaving the surgical debate we met an intern who engulfed us in a nightmare of unhappiness. He was caring for a sixteen-year-old girl who was dying from cystic fibrosis. Her lungs were plugged full of mucus and ravaged with pneumonia. No therapeutic reserves were left to throw into the struggle. The child would probably die in a matter of hours. The big problem now was the father. He had broken under the stress of watching his daughter die. He was inconsolable and had threatened to jump from the hospital roof as soon as she died.

The usual steps had been taken. The nurses and the intern had talked to the social workers. A psychiatrist had visited the father, but he was refusing all offers of help. No one could reach through his vision of celestial injustice. The intern was frightened.

"What should I do tonight if she dies, and he runs off the floor, screaming about suicide?"

Dr. Sanders frowned. "There's not much you can do. Call security, I guess, and tell them your fears. I hate to say it, but we have to protect the hospital." He paused. "I know it sounds callous, but there are limits to our responsibilities. At some point people take actions that are beyond our influence. It is the father's horrible duty to deal with this tragedy. Pete, it's not your problem. It's his."

This hard-nosed but honest advice troubled me all evening. About eleven o'clock, no longer able to concentrate on my books, I slipped out for a beer at a local tavern. Over a glass of Guiness I thought about the dying girl and her father. The story went round and round in my mind, but I could draw no conclusions. It seemed perfectly unfair.

A burst of cold air and familiar voices broke my somber reverie. The largest group of medical students I had ever seen assembled outside of a lecture hall had descended upon my private haunt. Clearly, some sort of madness had engulfed the dormitory where most of the class lived. Flushed faces and disheveled clothes made the diagnosis easy: The freshman class was on its first group bender. It was impossible to refuse; I joined them for a second glass. But the black thoughts kept lurking. Less than a mile away a man was pacing the fourth floor of the hospital, planning his own death. Try as I might I could not integrate this image with the raucous, happy scene that swirled about me. How could these events possibly be simultaneous?

As if he could read minds, Dr. Sanders told us the denouement of this tragedy as soon as we met on the following Thursday.

"The little girl with cystic fibrosis died last Saturday. Her father took it badly. He is in the neuropsychiatric unit now. Any other follow-ups? OK. I've got some great patients for us to meet today."

In early November a second clinical tutorial program started. Some fourth-year students had volunteered to shepherd us through the first bumbling attempts to take a "history." After seven or eight afternoons with Dr. Sanders this word had filtered into my vocabulary, but, as I donned my new white coat and hurried off to meet my senior tutor, I realized that I actually had no idea how to conduct a history. What questions were you supposed to ask? In what order? What answers were normal? I had not the slightest idea of how to interview a patient.

John, a thickly set ex-college tackle and one of the most talkative men I have ever met, took me and two classmates in tow. He had arranged for us to visit a patient named Mrs. Haller, a fifty-year-old woman who had been admitted to the hospital to undergo a cardiac catheterization. For forty minutes we listened while John asked her an unending series of questions about the chest pain that she felt when she exercised. From there he moved to questions about her past medical history, her family life, and her social history. The last subject he raised was whether she had any questions about the "heart test" that she would undergo in the morning. She had none.

This was the first of thousands of patient histories that I would witness in my life, so I was very eager to monitor my own impressions. As the questions shifted away from medically safe subjects like pain to more intimate questions about her family, I began to feel extremely uncomfortable, almost as though I were a "peeping Tom." Why should she be asked to unlock the secrets of her family life for me? It could not possibly be relevant to her illness, or could it? Her jovial manner and the ease with which she told her story made me all the more confused. A second observation that really troubled me was her apparent lack of concern for her illness. This lady was going to have a catheter threaded into her heart in the morning, yet she seemed completely relaxed. Did she realize the gravity of her illness? Had she been properly informed about the risks and benefits of cardiac catheterization? Or was she just a bit of flotsam caught up in the currents of medicine?

After the interview, John corralled us in a small room behind the nursing station. Right off, he challenged us to recount as much as we could remember about the history. We performed miserably.

"Train yourselves to listen," he urged. "You should have learned as much from that interview as I did. We heard exactly the same words." The next subject was "pain."

"How many times have you ever tried carefully to describe pain?"

"Never," we agreed. That was, after all, a task for the sick, and we were all healthy young adults.

"Start thinking about pain and discomfort. In eighteen months it will become the most important topic in your life. You are going to devote a lot of energy to deciphering what people mean when they talk about pain. Your life will be a lot easier if you develop ways to make sense out of the description that your patients offer."

"What's the secret?" cajoled a classmate.

"Everyone does it differently. I think of eight questions when I talk about pain: What brings it on? How long does it last? How often does it appear? What makes it worse? What makes it better? Where is it located? Does it radiate? How debilitating is it? You will develop your own way to ask these questions and others like them."

During Thanksgiving break I made a spectacle of myself by asking friends and family to describe their aches and pains. Other than learning that nearly everyone I knew was disgustingly healthy, I remained in the dark about the diagnostic arts.

On our first Thursday after Christmas break we found Dr. Sanders unusually tense. There had been an outbreak of meningitis. That afternoon we saw two children with "meningococcal meningitis." As Dr. Sanders told us how antibiotics had ended the meningococci's reign of terror, we grew steadily impressed. Just fifty years ago this disease killed almost nine out of ten victims; today mortality is less than 5 percent! As Dr. Sanders put it, the children we had seen today were not even sick enough "to earn a bed in the intensive care unit."

Perhaps stimulated by that remark, he next took us on our maiden voyage through the pediatric ICU (intensive care unit). It exceeded my wildest fantasies. In one corner lay a severely burned child. He looked like an actor who had been worked over by a bad makeup artist for a grade B horror flick. Great black scabs formed islands in a red sea of raw flesh that engulfed his face. His eyes were puffy and swollen shut. A nurse told me his brother had perished in the same fire that had erupted where a gas heater exploded in his ghetto tenement. A couple of beds away was a child in "status epilepticus." His little body writhed unceasingly, as though it were being hit with jolt after jolt of electricity.

Dr. Sanders explained that they were going to administer a dose of intravenous Valium—a drug that would stop his seizure but might further depress his ability to breathe. They would have to intubate him quickly. Try as I might, I could not imagine myself standing in the shoes of those residents.

In the far corner behind a curtain was a young, black teenage girl who was dying of fulminant hepatitis (liver failure). She was already comatose and her skin had a horrible purple-yellow hue. This time the jaundice was unmistakable. She lay face-up, her head entwined by the plastic tubing that carried the oxygen from her respirator to the "trach" tube jutting from her neck. She was naked, so Dr. Sanders stopped to teach us how to palpate a liver. One by one we each stood over this comatose teenager and probed her abdomen with stiffened fingers to feel the prominent liver edge.

She was jaundiced, comatose, and dying, but this was the first time I had confronted a naked young woman in a hospital bed, and her sexuality overpowered me. The dark nipples on her small, beautiful breasts were turgid. Her flat, firm belly flared out to a woman's hips. As I gazed at her it flashed through my mind that all over America men flock to "topless" bars to mix a little voyeurism with their alcohol. I bent forward to press my fingers into her belly, to rub the edge of her swollen liver. I realized that probably the only men who had ever touched her breasts were the doctors who were watching her die. I wondered what dreams she had had of boyfriends, lovers, a husband, and children. A miasma descended; I was lost in a confused jumble as images of sex and death, unfamiliar partners, danced together. Adolescence is a particularly cruel time to die; life should not be snatched away just as dreams are beginning to take root and flower.

After our first visit to the pediatric ICU, Dr. Sanders made it a standard part of our Thursday afternoon

rounds—as though he had decided to teach us about
tragedy. On the last day of January this education reached
new heights. The senior resident was about to disconnect
the respirator that was breathing for a fifteen-year-old boy
with a battered skull. He lay propped up in the first bed,
his well-muscled body and handsome face belying that he
was not merely napping. But his brain was dead, pulver-
ized when his skidding sled darted in front of a truck. Dr.
Sanders drew us to the bedside, shut off the overhead
light, and gently pushed apart his eyelids. He blasted a ray
of bright light into his right eye, but it was unyielding. The
pupil did not constrict. The brain was unaware of light; it
was no longer processing information.

The intern and resident were hunched over styrofoam
cups of coffee at the nursing station. The intern was
furious. He had been caring for a dead patient for a week,
while the parents struggled to accept the horrible truth
that they had lost a son. It had been less than an hour since
they had finally agreed that the respirator should be disconnected. Now it was merely a matter of waiting until a
surgical team was assembled to harvest the boy's kidneys.
The senior resident waited until the intern had vented his
feelings, then joined us.

"We see a lot of death here," he admitted. "It is not too
hard to accept the death of a newborn with a severe birth
defect. Nobody, not even the parents, gets too attached to
a baby like that. It has been hard, but I have even learned
to accept the deaths of children from leukemia. These are
hard, but a lot of mourning gets done in advance, and there
is a strange logic to disease.

"But death because of an automobile accident sickens
me. It is more senseless than war. It is very, very hard. For
these parents, especially, it was nearly impossible."

He told us the family's tale. The boy's father was a
psychologist who directed a home for the mentally retarded. He had been drawn to this work after one son had

been born with Down's syndrome, a form of mental retardation. The second of his three children had also suffered severe developmental problems. The family's dreams had ridden on the shoulders of their only healthy son. The story drained me. I was numb. Surely, it could not be true. But denial did not work here; I had only to turn my head to see the boy entangled in IV tubing and guarded by monitors. For the first of many times in medical school I thought of the story of Job. What kind of world was I entering?

One February afternoon the clinical correlations conference was devoted to "heart sounds." The entire class assembled in Fitkin Amphitheater, hoping that a prominent physician who was nicknamed "The Heart" would dispel the overwhelming sense of mystery that descended whenever we placed a stethoscope to a chest. He had a neat teaching scheme. Each of us was given a "stethophone," an instrument that looked like a cross between a stethoscope and a telephone jack. After plugging the jacks into their sockets beneath the chairs in the lecture hall we could commune with Dr. Henshaw's special toy, a "heart sound simulator." Under his fatherly guidance we plugged ourselves in, and he taught us the components of the heart sounds, like a piano master teaching kindergarten.

Within moments the blanket of fog began to lift. Henshaw taught us how to catch hold of the first heart sound (by timing the intervals between the two beats) and to feel out its rate and rhythm. By twirling the dials of his magic machine he could give us a heart that beat slowly and majestically sixty times a minute. To the human ear, which can discern sounds that are separated by only thirty milliseconds, a second is a very long time. Even a beginner can time the rate and distinguish the two heart sounds. After five minutes at this speed I was feeling a great sense of relief. But then Dr. Henshaw increased the rate to eighty ("the speed of a healthy adult's heart as he walks down the street") and then to one hundred ("a mild tachycardia"). At eighty I could still follow the pattern, but at the higher rate all order disappeared. I heard only an unending succession of muffled knocks by an impatient delivery boy at the front door. Then "The Heart" turned the dial to one hundred and twenty, "the normal pace of a baby's heart." Matters grew worse. How could anyone ever hear a murmur hidden between these sounds? After he had disconnected the heart sound simulator, the master, reading the confusion in our faces wrought by his fearful machine, gave us a fatherly pep talk.

"Don't worry about high-speed heart sounds," he reassured us. "If you could distinguish any two heart sounds at any speed, you have the ears to be a cardiologist. It is all a matter of practice. See you on the wards."

Week after week Dr. Sanders brought another medical "first" into our lives. In early March we went to an M&M (morbidity and mortality) conference. This is a weekly meeting at which the surgeons and other physicians discuss the treatment of patients who had serious complications or deaths during or after surgery. We went because they were going to discuss a child for whom Dr. Sanders had cared—a little girl with ulcerative colitis. This mysterious, chronic inflammation of the colon often requires a bowel resection. After the child had undergone surgery to remove a piece of her bowel, she had developed a fistula, a communication between the inside of the body and the skin, a tunnel from the operative site, that would not heal.

I had barely settled into a plush seat in the back row of the surgical conference room when I felt the tension in the atmosphere. An aggressive, sword-wielding surgeon, the man who had done the bowel resection, was attacking a quiet, scholarly radiologist because one of his residents had allegedly misinterpreted a key x-ray film. The pediatricians hugged the sidelines, watching the carnage. The surgeon simply would not let the radiologist reply. Only after ranting and raving for five minutes did he concede the floor. From the large group of surgeons, a frozen skepticism greeted the radiologist's careful explanation of why the film had been so difficult to read. The surgeons reminded me of jet pilots reviewing the failure of a bombing run. Convinced that their mission had failed because a support service had let them down, they were not going to change their minds. I walked out of the room with a knot in my stomach; I just did not thrive in such a hostile climate!

Anxiety is a constant feature of medical students' lives. As months slip away and students begin to grasp the dimensions of their ignorance, the anxiety flowers. As they begin to see patients, the abyss that separates their competence from that of "real" doctors widens. Wearing a white coat, carrying a stethoscope, seeing patients, medical students look like doctors and patients address them as such. Many teachers introduce them as part of the medical team. In their fantasy lives they already are great healers. Lying in bed late at night, they ease the suffering of a cancer patient or perform heroic surgery. But walking the wards or talking with patients is a different matter. They are acutely aware they are not doctors. Indeed, this goal sometimes seems to be receding despite forward progress through medical school. For not a few people the anxiety becomes particularly painful whenever they are introduced to patients with the word *doctor*. It is difficult to know whether this discomfort is caused by a genuine ethical concern that patients are being misinformed or (as I suspect) by students' intense feelings of incompetence.

I was not surprised to learn one April afternoon that a group called the Conference on Health and Human Values had planned a forum to consider the question, Should medical students be introduced to patients as doctors? These conferences were not usually well attended, but by four o'clock Fitkin Amphitheater was overfull. Obviously, a lot of other people had anxiety about this question.

A student from each of the first-, second-, and third-year classes spoke. All agreed that to introduce a student as a "doctor" to a patient violated a fundamental principle of truth-telling. As the presentations proceeded, the arguments grew more insistent. But only the first-year student admitted that the title embarrassed him. The keynote speaker was Dr. Joseph Conally, a psychiatrist who had written much about informed consent. Dr. Conally answered the question with what he described as a "tentative no." "In medicine," he warned, "one must be constantly vigilant to avoid the traps of self-delusion."

The audience, which included many fourth-year students (lame ducks waiting to graduate), seemed to disagree with many of the speaker's points.

"Getting a diploma does not make you a doctor," argued one. "When you are directly involved in the act of caring for a person and making treatment decisions in his behalf, then you are a doctor. These are things that third-year students do."

"Don't worry," admonished another. "You will feel quite comfortable with the 'doctor' label by the second on-call night of your subinternship." (Subinternship—when the student works on a floor for six weeks and takes direct responsibility for patient care—is the crowning clinical experience of medical school.) Knowing laughter danced through the crowd.

"If you are motivated by compassion, you should not allow yourself to be defeated by ignorance," argued a third. "If you are caring for a patient, it is wrong *not* to call yourself a doctor," he persisted.

I walked out of the hall feeling hopeful. Something had happened to those fourth-year students along the way. They had come to terms with at least some of their anxiety.

On the last Thursday in April we met with Dr. Sanders for the last time. He had arranged for us to observe heart surgery on a little baby. It was our first trip to an operating room, and it could not have been made more impressive if the scene had been planned in Hollywood. We began in the observation room, a small glassed-in overhang that looked down onto the OR. The OR was large, perhaps the dimension of an elegant living room in an expensive home. The walls were plaster and the floor was squares of black tile flecked with white. Large glass cabinets filled with suture sets, instruments, and drugs lined two walls. The room was jammed. There were five people bent over the baby at the table, and nine others were stationed elsewhere. After a few minutes one of the nine looked up, waved to Dr. Sanders, and came to us.

The mask fell away to reveal a tough-looking woman named Janice Mowry, a pediatric cardiologist. She tried to explain the infant's problem, a rare condition called "cor triatrium biventriculum," but as her approach was to ask us questions about cardiac function that I could not answer, she succeeded only in intimidating me. Next she divided us into pairs and brought each pair into the OR, admonishing us to do "exactly what I say." Never have I seen such perfect obedience. We were terrified of disrupting this dramatic scene.

A tiny infant, weighing ten pounds, was the object of this attention. He had been placed on a heart-lung machine. His body temperature had been cooled greatly, and his circulatory needs were being controlled by a squat boxlike machine that stood fifteen feet from his heart. It reminded me of an old ice chest on top of which stood two glass containers shaped like jars of mayonnaise into which connected clear plastic tubes red with blood. This system included a filter that removed the carbon dioxide and reoxygenated the baby's blood.

Dr. Mowry led me to a stool next to the anesthesiologist at the head of the table. From this vantage point I could look over the shoulders of the surgeons. Wearing special helmets with powerful miner's lights and jeweler's lenses that could be flipped down by a nurse, these men looked more like lunar explorers than doctors. I was amazed at the tiny perimeter within which they worked. This operation was being done through an incision of only two inches.

We passed most of the afternoon in and about the OR. When Dr. Sanders led us to the locker room to change back into street clothes I thought we had finished. "It's only four-thirty," he said. "I've got one more thing to show you." Over the year we had become familiar with his taciturn nature; rather than ask questions, we just sailed along in his wake. It was a long walk through the oldest part of the hospital to a corner which I had not yet visited. Only when I saw that a short side corridor was lined with ancient gurneys (stretchers on wheels) did I realize we were going to end our clinical tutorial at the morgue.

The old green-tiled room was suitably quiet. The six steel tables were shiny-clean and there was not a pathologist in sight. The place seemed closed down for the night. Dr. Sanders pointed to the table at the farthest corner.

"There's what I am looking for."

A small white plastic bag lay over a tiny mound in the table's center. As we approached and I saw the head, my first, involuntary, thought was, "Somebody left a doll down here." Even after Dr. Sanders had drawn away the sheet, it took me a moment to digest the ineluctable fact that a newly dead infant lay before me. The child was very beautiful; blond hair and long eyelashes gave her a cherubic look. Only her pale cheeks and perfect stillness spoke of death.

No one said a word. I wondered if Ron and Neal and
James were thinking what I was thinking. This baby did not
belong all alone on this cold table in a hospital cellar. It was
not fair. I felt very uncomfortable. Until now my commu-
nion with human death had been through the dissection of
a cadaver that had been pickled in brine for two years while
he waited my arrival. Even before we had dismembered
him, he had lost a lot of his human look. This beautiful
infant would surely cry if I picked her up and shook her
awake. I stepped back from the table. On a nearby counter
I spied a large steel basin. In it lay a blackened, scarred
human lung, gelled in clots of its own blood. The contrast
to the infant's purity was startling. For a fleeting moment I
feared that Dr. Sanders had brought us to witness an
autopsy. This was too horrible. I could not watch somebody
carve up that baby.

A moment later Sanders broke the silence: "This little
girl died today of something very strange that we call
sudden infant death syndrome. It is just a phrase to
describe something we do not understand. I thought you
should see her. I always wonder how such a healthy looking
infant can be dead. Maybe one of you guys will figure it out
someday." He paused. "Let's go."

We saw Dr. Sanders once more that year. Over beer and
pizza we reminisced for an hour and then gave him a small
gift. I saw him only a few times during the rest of my stay at
Yale, but his face still flashes through my mind whenever I
encounter something new in medicine.

Chapter 3

PATHOLOGY

My first year of medical education ended a few weeks after my last session with Dr. Sanders. Although each course offered a final examination, at Yale one could (and the majority did) take them anonymously. The relative unimportance of tests made the end of the year much more tolerable, but it deprived us of a milestone. Instead of meeting together in the lecture hall one last time, people faded into the lilac softness of late May. Especially for those of us who did not live in the dormitory, there were relatively few good-byes. They did not seem particularly necessary. After all, September would find the same 102 people assembled for the third (and final) semester of classroom education.

The summer after the first year of medical school is the only one that is not officially part of the curriculum. Although various officials urged us to spend this time researching our thesis (a requirement almost unique to Yale), many of us perceived these three months to be a last taste of freedom. Not surprisingly, the range of summer activities was wide. Some students worked ten or twelve hours a day in research labs; others, hoping to pare the huge burden of medical school tuition, worked at whatever jobs they could get, and a few just loafed. Unlike the quiet anxiety of the first, the second September found us sitting in a familiar room surrounded by friendly faces. For the moment, at least, we could bask in the self-assurance of being seasoned veterans. There was now a class behind us that craved our advice.

Three great courses dominated the third semester of medical school: microbiology, pharmacology, and pathology. The microbiology course introduced us to the tiny killers that had tormented physicians for centuries. Each afternoon the lecturers spun yet another Homeric tale of the exploits of physicians in the bacterial wars. Not so many decades ago, the innocent-looking diplococci, dancing in pairs on my slide, had easily killed young and old. Penicillin had ended that reign of terror. One afternoon I looked through a "dark-field" microscope at the sensual, writhing *Treponema pallidum*. Until World War II, syphilis, the legacy left by this curvy spirochete, was rivaled only by tuberculosis as the most devastating disease in the West. Now, syphilis was a trivial therapeutic problem. There were also newer victories. One day a professor explained the molecular biology by which cholera dehydrated people to death, and convinced us that despite its deadly reputation this organism would not be able to kill any person who could be given adequate fluids and nursing care. The microbiology course recited a wonderful litany of victories by physicians over disease. This was heady stuff.

Pharmacology was equally exciting. The Department of Pharmacology at Yale was one of the strongest in the world. These men were scientific titans, whose research had fostered new understanding about the interaction of chemicals with cells and had led to the development of new drugs. Day after day one could walk out of the lecture hall amazed at the beautiful symmetry with which the world was organized. Why was it that a world in which people died from the havoc of tiny bacteria was also the home of penicillin and streptomycin, molds that easily exploded killer bugs but gently ignored human cells? The study of the nitrogen mustards, chemicals that had burned the lungs of thousands of soldiers in the trenches of World War I, had led to the development of the first effective agents against cancer! How wonderful that William Withering, a simple country doctor, had noticed the bizarre connection between the foxglove weed and the sudden improvement of an old lady with congestive heart failure. By boiling the weed and drinking judiciously of its juice, one could cure cardiac asthma. Digitalis, one of our most important heart medicines, is just essence of foxglove!

The most exciting course of all was pathology; it was here that the darkest secrets of disease were revealed. Other courses spoke of victories, but pathology told of defeats and battles still to be fought. Were these not the most important things to know? The vast course was divided into four parts: an unending series of lectures, a laboratory devoted to the microscopic examination of tissue devastated by illness, a second laboratory devoted to the examination of the whole organs that had been riddled by disease and deformity, and a weekly seminar in which professors met with us in small groups to analyze particular problems.

The histopathology laboratory began on an enticing note. The first session was designed to illustrate one of the most basic defense mechanisms that protect the human body: the inflammatory response. Since ancient times physicians had observed "rubor, calor, dolor, and tumor," the redness, heat, pain, and swelling that followed local injury. The microscope permitted us to watch the cellular basis of this phenomenon. One day we learned something that the mad Russian pathologist Menchnikoff had discovered in a classic experiment a century ago. An anesthetized white mouse lay on a scaffold by the microscope. Under the lens his delicate, translucent pink ear resolved into highways of arterioles, capillaries, and venules. A single scratch had been made with a needle. Traffic was very busy, but near the scratch it looked like rush hour. In the center lane red blood cells hurried home from work, angrily weaving around the larger leukocytes. These white blood cells were up to something. As they approached the injured area they seemed to pull out of the center lane to the highway's shoulder.

There they bumped and jostled against the vessel walls. Outside the vessels were an extraordinary number of white cells at the site of injury, resembling ambulances near the scene of a terrible accident. Somehow the white cells had been able to slip through the vessel walls to get to the scene. They could now hunt and kill any bacteria that had sneaked through the break in the skin made by the scratch. This phenomenon is called "margination" because leukocytes seemed to line the edge of the vessels before exiting. Fantastic!

Although there were a few other dramatic demonstrations during the semester, the vast majority of our time in histopathology was spent poring over the "teaching slides" from the slotted wooden boxes that we had been loaned. Each of the cracked old slides with yellowed labels offered a classic picture of the devastation heaped on a particular tissue by a particular disease. For reasons completely unknown to me, I remember one slide with special clarity: Kimmelstiel-Wilson disease—a fancy eponym for the effects that severe diabetes can have on the kidney. The nephron is the basic structural element of the kidney. The two million nephrons with which we are born constitute an incredible conservation system that saves valuable chemicals and flushes out the body's poisons. Every day, year in and year out, the kidneys filter about 5000 quarts of blood (of course, the body contains only five quarts of blood, but it is pumped around and around all day long), removing and excreting all the wastes as a single quart of urine and recirculating the rest. The efficiency with which it maintains blood volume and excretes poisons is nothing less than incredible.

The crucial first step in filtration occurs at the glomerulus, a beautiful tuft of vessels and specialized cells attached to a long, looping tube, like a delicate undersea plant swaying in unseen currents. Nestled in a "Bowman's" capsule, the specialized cells at the end of the stalk filter the blood's "water." Through its long journey down the proximal tubule, through the hairpin loop of Henle and out the distal tubule to the collection system, and ultimately to the bladder, this water is constantly filtered by a vast array of special cells. We can lose many, indeed most, of our glomeruli without being aware of any disturbance in our health, but if too many die, disaster ensues. If the filtering process falls even slightly behind the demands placed upon it by the other trillions of cells, the body succumbs rapidly to chemical pollution. For failing kidneys the alternatives are simple: a kidney transplant, chronic dialysis, or uremic death.

In Kimmelstiel-Wilson disease the basement membrane, a crucial structure of the cells in the glomerulus, is melted by diabetes. The microscope shows that the organization of the normal glomerulus is extremely delicate and distinct. One can pick out the vessels, the mesangial cells, and the other special cells that perform the vital filtration. In contrast, the glomerulus of someone with this disorder is just a smudge of pink stain. With the microscope set at low power one can survey a large section of kidney and see the roundish smudges of pink scattered throughout the cross-section of normal-looking tubules and support tissues. It was like looking down from an airplane at the puffs of smoke billowing up from a field after a fire. The destruction was everywhere. I shall never forget this convincing slide.

Two mornings a week our first task was the study of "specimens." About 8:05 the first of twenty bleary-eyed medical students would shuffle into the third-floor lab, trying not to contaminate their take-out coffee and rolls with any of the disgusting objects piled on the low black tables. No matter how tardy the students, the pathology resident always seemed to arrive last. The only obvious difference between him and us was the unconcern about where he placed his daily fare of two jelly doughnuts.

Specimen is a polite term. Each morning we faced different mounds of gray-brown organs that recalled an ancient baseball glove that my collie had once stolen and chewed for three days. They smelled worse than they looked. Our job in this lab was to move from table to table examining several dozen of these objects, guess what horror their previous owner had suffered, and then read the correct diagnosis, which was printed neatly on a tag wrapped by wire to each. This was not at all easy. Often it took the full force of my creative powers to guess which organ it was, let alone identify the particular "lesion," as our resident fondly called them. Several decades in jars of formaldehyde gave a curious oneness to hearts and kidneys. I distinctly remember the morning a visiting professor pointed out an enlarged prostate that on closer examination turned out to be a child's small uterus. This somewhat reassured me!

At the specimen laboratory, attendance peaked quickly and fell off rapidly. By 9:15 only six or seven hardy souls were left. The pathology lecture did not start until ten, so, unless I had opted to join a colleague in a long coffee break, I dutifully examined specimen after specimen. The most instructive organs were the hearts with congenital defects. When one poked a finger through a VSD (a hole in the heart's middle wall) or ran a probe through a patent ductus (a persistent remnant of fetal life), open heart surgery took on new meaning. The livers and lungs that were loaded with cancer were also especially dramatic. The sound of the word *cancer* took on a new ugliness as I examined livers swollen with tumors the size of baseballs and lungs glued to tracheas by adenocarcinomas.

My faculty seminar was directed by a rather pedantic woman who had spent twenty years investigating the causes of cardiomyopathy—studying why some hearts dilate, become floppy, and stop working. We met every Wednesday afternoon in her impossibly cluttered and overheated office to hold a CPC (clinical-pathological conference). One of the great traditions in medicine, the CPC was refined as a teaching device over a century ago at the Massachusetts General Hospital. It always begins with a full narrative description of a patient's illness. A physician then considers the patient's differential diagnosis, and rationally narrows the possibilities to a final diagnosis. The pathologist, blessed with the certainty of hindsight, then gives the correct analysis based on his or her microscope work.

The CPC is one of the most effective teaching techniques in medical education, but it also is a deadly intellectual game. Physicians delight in seeing a famous colleague stumped by a CPC, especially if it ends up in the pages of a medical journal. On the other hand, some of the most astute clinicians seem almost unstumpable. One bit of Yale folklore involves a young professor of medicine who was reputed to be a diagnostic genius. He once accepted the invitation of a rival medical school to lead a CPC. As was customary, he received the patient narrative a few days in advance. The story was impenetrable: A completely healthy thirty-year-old man with no medical history had collapsed and died a few hours after returning to Los Angeles from an uneventful vacation in Amsterdam. The deck had been stacked against him, but the Yale professor nevertheless played his hand. The conference was unusually crowded that day, and he watched the smiles of his peers broaden as the size of his differential diagnosis increased rather than narrowed. At the end he had considered everything from heart attack to spider bite. Just as he seemed about to admit defeat, his tone changed to one of utter confidence and he proclaimed, "I believe that this case permits only one diagnosis. This man died after several packets of heroin that he had swallowed in attempting to sneak through customs burst in his stomach." The applause proved that the diagnosis was correct!

One late October day while I was drifting through an abstruse immunology lecture on the intricacies of T-cell suppression, I was jolted to attention by the sound of my own name. The secretary of the Department of Pathology was standing by the lectern. Dr. McClellan, the hotshot young immunologist who looked like a clone of Leon Trotsky, was holding a note as he repeated the call.

"Mr. Reilly? Is Mr. Reilly here?"

"Yes, sir." I waved my hand.

"They want you downstairs."

A low chuckle drifted through the class. I rose grimly. It was my turn to attend an autopsy.

Hurrying along the dimly lit basement corridors to the morgue, I remembered a story that Dr. Frost had recounted about Leonardo da Vinci, one of the greatest anatomists in history. Da Vinci procured his cadavers from a monastery that offered shelter to destitute old people. He was friendly with many of the monks, especially a most ancient man who was reputed to have celebrated one hundred birthdays. Leonardo was fascinated that this spry old monk still rose at dawn to work the gardens. One day he heard that the monk had been found dead in his cell. He immediately petitioned the abbot for permission to perform an autopsy, a request that he had never before made about the body of a brother of the Church. The abbot was troubled by this request and asked why Leonardo wished to subject a holy man to a procedure reserved for thieves and beggars. "I study the dead to learn how men may live well," said Leonardo. "Surely, God has hidden the secret of the good life in this man's body."

Probably no other exercise has contributed as much to human health as the autopsy. Beginning with the golden age of anatomy in Italy five centuries ago when Vesalius first dared to dissect systematically the remains of executed criminals, the autopsy has revealed the dark secrets of disease. In the mid-nineteenth century the great German pathologists, led by Virchow, turned pathology into a science. Armed with knives, microscopes, and burning curiosity, in three extraordinary decades they discovered our modern notions of how diseases kill. The greatest advances in the treatment of disease were made by the doctors who mastered pathology. William Osler, a legendary physician who worked at Johns Hopkins School of Medicine at the turn of the century, claimed that the time he spent at the dissecting table (as a young man he performed a thousand autopsies) was the most valuable of his life.

Twenty-five years ago the autopsy was still a dominant feature of the pathology course. For example, at one major state school second-year medical students were required to observe twenty, assist in dissection at ten, and write up five autopsies. Caught now in the revolution that carries us deeper into the world of subcellular elements and molecular bases of disease, the student's attention is pulled to electron microscopy and radioimmunoassays. Each year the autopsy table yields more time. At Yale, students are barely exposed to autopsies, and many graduate having stood at the table only once. I had different intentions.

The morgue door was open. An old, wizened black man hunched over a magazine at a scarred wooden desk in a corner office. He was the diener, the man who handled the bodies before and after the doctors did their work, the man who stuffed in the organs, stitched the body back together, and hosed away the bile and blood. No one could be more familiar with death. The morgue was a single large room with apple-green walls and wooden shelves that ran nearly to the ceiling. Hundreds of large glass jars, each holding the culprit that had caused the demise of persons now long dead, lined the shelves. The far end of the room was a wall of human brains, making the morgue look like a ghoulish supermarket at the edge of the River Styx.

An old-fashioned, deeply scalloped ceramic sink beckoned from one corner. I rolled up my sleeves, washed my hands, and donned a white plastic apron no thicker than Saran Wrap—a very fragile barrier between me and death, but at least it would stop the blood. I pulled on a pair of cheap latex gloves and joined the resident at the stone table. He was a big guy named Dan who greeted me with a warm smile and a slow Virginia drawl.

"I'm new at this," he said. "John here," he patted the dead man's shoulder, "is my sixteenth. I'll be moving slowly, but maybe that's better for you," he paused. "I know they make you guys come down here. Are you at all interested?"

"Don't worry about me, Dan. I'm interested."

"Fine. I'll teach you what I can. Why don't you start by telling me what you see, while I sharpen this knife."

If I had learned one thing from pathology, it was the crucial importance of recognizing the patently obvious. I slowly inspected the corpse, trying to record every impression as my eyes slid from his bald pate to his horny, broken toenails.

"On the table in front of us is a thin white male, looking well over seventy years of age. He has a surgical scar on the right upper side of his abdomen. The most impressive thing I see is a cupcake-shaped lump beneath the skin by his right collarbone. There is a cardboard tag tied to his right big toe that lists his name, age, and hospital number."

"Good. Do you know what that lump is?"

"No."

"That is a pacemaker. That means that this old boy had a bad ticker. Not too surprising at his age, is it? A faulty pacemaker can explain a cardiac death. Our first job will be to remove that device and its wires as neatly as possible. We'll describe it, then we will send it to the pacemaker lab for analysis."

He picked up a small, curved knife, and quickly inscribed a semicircle around the lump's lower border. The blood, clotted by death, looked like curds of grape jelly. He folded back the skin and fat to uncover the shiny metal object with two thin wires burrowing toward the heart. These he removed with a firm tug. I wondered silently if this was good technique. What if death had been caused by a dislodged wire? Having removed the pacemaker, he picked up a larger, thicker blade that looked as though it could decapitate a cow, and set to work. The first cuts ran from the points of the shoulders to the top of the breast bone. After he had formed that V, he made a long straight steady incision right to the pubic hair. The famous autopsy Y was completed.

"Now you can help. Pick up the skin and retract it for me while I flay him."

In seconds the skin lay in two flaps draped over each arm, and the ribs glistened. Oozing blood gave a sheen to the healthy-looking red muscles.

"This part doesn't take much brains, just brawn. Now we have to cut and remove the entire rib cage in one piece."

Ten minutes later, after hacking away with a bone shears and knives, the ribs lay like the shield of a Mayan warrior on the thighs of his vanquished foe. A steady trickle of blood curled through the smooth sheet of cold water that ran from the upwardly tilted head of the table to the drain beneath the dead man's feet. Deprived of their protective ribs, his lungs and heart lay defenseless before us. The muscular diaphragm and large blood vessels still anchored them firmly in place. Below it, more colorful and dramatic than the best drawing, were the liver and stomach, the omental curtain with its lumps of butter-yellow fat, and a mass of wormy intestines. In thirty seconds I learned more about the spatial relationships of the abdominal organs than I had grasped in months of anatomy. A cadaver's organs are all mousy gray, and we had so thoroughly dismembered each section of Kojak that it had been impossible to appreciate the big picture.

The next task was to remove the heart, lungs, and great vessels in a single block. After carefully inspecting the organ surfaces, Dan took a tiny scimitar and transected the trachea and the descending aorta, and dissected away various adhesions (scar tissue) that anchored the lungs to the body wall. With a deft twist he yanked out lungs and heart and held them at arm's length, as they dripped over the table. Turning to a smaller wooden slab he separated the three organs. Next, he weighed them on an old-fashioned butcher's scale that hung from the ceiling. As he called out the weights, I recorded them on the autopsy sheet. The empty chest cavity now looked like the interior of an artfully carved canoe, a masterpiece of some primitive pygmy culture.

Turning to the abdomen, Dan again quickly inspected each organ. A small, green, scarred gallbladder peeked out from beneath the liver.

"Feel that gall bag," he ordered, "and describe it to me."

"Stones," I said. "It feels like dozens of tiny stones."

"You're a born pathologist," he kidded.

The big surprise came when we explored the left upper quadrant. As he reflected the pancake-shaped spleen to the left and I pulled the bowels toward the feet, a platoon of "accessory spleens" marched into view. Proceeding from the main spleen toward the midline we counted six extra organs, ranging in size from a clam shell to a pea. This was an unusual finding: Only one in four hundred people had extra spleens.

"Let's not jump the gun," cautioned Dan. "Those could be large lymph nodes. We'll have to wait for the microscope's opinion."

The next job was to "run the bowel." Dan double-clamped the duodenum (the part of the small intestine that connects to the stomach, the great C-shaped section seen well in old Pepto-Bismol ads). Then he made a long cut into the stomach wall. I felt slightly sick. This man had dined on white rice, salad, and chicken for his last meal. Scooping out the half-processed food, we inspected the rugae, the complex, delicate folds of mucosa that contain millions of cells, each a special chemical factory. The rugae reminded me of a satellite photo of a rugged mountain range.

The small bowel lay like a tangle of pale garden snakes before us. The intestines are firmly rooted to the body's back wall by the mesentery. After clamping the large bowel close to the rectum, Dan started cutting the intestines away from the mesenteric stalk. The plan was to lift the entire bowel mass out in one loop, immerse it in a tub of water, and "milk out" the feces. I was trying to figure out the scientific rationale for this maneuver when disaster struck. Dan nicked the descending colon. There was a long, slow hiss of gas. Seconds later I was hit by the worst stench I have ever smelled. Only my bloody gloves kept me from pinching my nose. I barely controlled the twin impulses to retch and run. A wave of hydrogen sulphide, methane, cadaverine, and a dozen other vapors swept over a pair of residents working at a nearby table.

"Dan, you idiot, did you cut his bowels?" moaned one.

"Take it easy, Andrew," cautioned another. "Maybe the medical student farted."

"Sorry, boys," grinned Dan. "It wasn't the stud. I confess."

Once the bowels were excised, we dumped them into a big metal tub. Picking up the northern end, Dan ran it through his fingers as though he were trying to straighten a curled ribbon. Unformed feces oozed steadily into the clouding water.

"This is nothing special. We just clean out the intestines so we can get a good look at the mucosal surface later on during our formal organ review. Most of the real work gets done with the microscope."

After he had finished this odd cleaning job, Dan put the intestines into a basin of clean water, and we turned back to the corpse.

"The best way to do any autopsy is to remove all parts of a system at once," he said. "So our next job is tricky. We have to harvest both kidneys, the ureters [the pipes that carry urine to the bladder], and the bladder. It's hard to avoid cutting or tearing the ureters. After I free up the beans [kidneys], we'll each try to dissect a ureter."

"OK."

The urinary tract is in the retroperitoneum. This means that it is lodged behind the layers of tissue that house the other abdominal organs. Because a frontal approach would trap the surgeon in a deep hole with poor exposure, kidney surgery is performed through a flank incision. Of course, the pathologist, who removes organs as he or she works, has little trouble with the frontal approach. But the kidney is buried in a depression and packed with fat, and the ureters run a curvy course to the bladder. It is easy to remove them, but it is not easy to remove them neatly.

Dan needed about fifteen minutes to pry the kidneys loose from the clutches of the perinephric fat. After that we identified the ureters. They looked like two greyish-white lengths of rubbery cord that ran parallel to the spine before plugging into the back of the bladder. Leaving about a quarter-inch on each side, we outlined their paths with our knives. That done, Dan quickly cut the bladder away from its adherent tissue. Together we laid the intact organs on an empty steel tray.

"Look at the upper pole of the right kidney. What do you see?"

"There's an area shaped like a slice of pie that's dark and sunken."

"Right. What's that?"

"We haven't studied kidneys much," I lamely answered.

"That's probably an infarct. A branch of one of the lobular arteries must have gotten clogged. That wedge of the kidney may have been dead for years."

Back to the table.

"I hate this part. We've got to cut off his balls. They, sad to say, get old and sick, too."

Dan slit the scrotum wide open and removed both testes.

"No obvious tumors." He tossed the testicles into the growing pile of organs. "Now for the nitty-gritty. Let's get to his brain."

He opened a gray metal box the size of a suburban tool kit and pulled out a cucumber-shaped object with an electric cord. It was a cast-cutting saw—a high-speed blade that could neatly divide the calvarium (the bony case that protects the brain). He plugged it in and flipped the toggle switch. The blade hummed. Satisfied that it was ready, Dan turned it off.

"First we have to scalp him. The trick is to be neat, so we don't catch hell from the funeral parlor. All they care about is the face."

The dead man's head rested on a small wooden block. I lifted it up so Dan could add a second block and push both under his neck. He took his sharpest knife, and starting just behind one ear, he drew a great semicircle through the hair to the other ear. Next he avulsed the scalp (a quarter-inch of skin and tough connective tissue) and peeled it forward to expose the crisp white skull. With the man's scalp hiding his face, and his entire skullcap exposed, the cast-cutting saw could do its work. Dan divided the calvarium with two even cuts that joined at the occiput (back of the head). With one hand he then lifted the bony cap and exposed the brain.

It sat snugly in its neat packing case, a grayish topographical mystery with dozens of smooth ridges that wandered off to nowhere. A narrow, deep crevice divided this strange object in two. At the bottom of the crevice hid the corpus callosum, the great crossroads that connected the right and left brains. A road map of tiny vessels crisscrossed these hills and valleys.

With his left hand Dan gently cupped the back of the brain and rocked it forward. In his right hand was a tiny scythe. He maneuvered it sideways between the brain and the skull and rotated it several times to transect the brain stem at the foramen magnum, the great hole at the base of the skull through which messages once raced to and from this body. This done, the rest was easy and the brain soon lay on a small steel tray, shivering with indignity.

"I'm getting hungry," Dan announced. "Let's quickly open the organs so you can see any obvious pathology. The formal organ review will be at four o'clock. Of course the microscope studies won't be ready until next week."

He picked up the heart and turned it over in his hands.

"There's a scarred area here," he pointed. "This man had an anterior wall MI [heart attack] some time ago. The scar tells me it's at least six months old, but it could also have happened twenty years ago. I don't see any obvious aneurysm, but this is a floppy, dilated heart. It could not have been working too well recently."

He slit open both ventricles. "Nothing too dramatic there. The little papillary muscles [they attach to the valves] are not ruptured. That's a quick way to die."

He split open the aorta and ran his gloved fingers along its gnarled surface. "Feel that tube. It's crooked and stiff and covered with warty plaques. This guy had the usual big-time atherosclerosis. Let's cut a coronary."

He made a small slice through the muscle to expose a cross-section of the left anterior descending artery, the "LAD" to cardiologists, the "widow-maker" to surgeons. Barely wider than the tip of a felt pen, the hollow center of the blood vessel was nearly closed off by cholesterol plaques. A section cut an inch away revealed the same thing. Not much room for blood.

"A setup for ischemic heart disease, but we can't say that killed him."

Next the lungs. They looked pretty good.

"I bet he never smoked," observed Dan.

He divided the great pulmonary artery, the vessel that brings used blood from the heart to be reoxygenated by the lungs. It was clean.

"I was looking for a saddle embolus. Blood clots can kill very quickly."

He surveyed the bowels.

"Let's look over the guts."

With a large bread knife, he lopped off a hunk of liver.

"Good architecture. Look at the sinusoids. Given what we've seen of this guy, I would have to put cancer low on my list. Liver metastases are really obvious. Of course, nearly everybody his age has cancer of the prostate, but that rarely kills you when you are eighty." He turned to the intestines. "The stomach and 'loops' also look pretty good. Say," he grinned, "maybe this guy isn't dead."

"What would you bet on?" I asked.

"Stroke. No blood to the brain."

I glanced at my watch. It was 12:50 and there was a

pharmacology lecture at one o'clock. I thanked Dan for his teaching and retreated to the cleanup sink. I added my soiled gloves and apron to the trash can. Miraculously, although I had forgotten to wear booties, my shoes were unstained. I scrubbed my hands and forearms, but ugly odors of death still danced in my nostrils. As I hurried out the door, I almost collided with the diener who was wheeling in another body. For now my inquisitiveness was quenched; I headed for sunshine.

The autopsy is one of the great passages in medical school. With the call to the morgue many students meet a newly dead body for the first time. The autopsy table is profoundly different from the anatomy table. Compared to a patient who has just died, an old pickled cadaver hardly seems human. All who have participated in an autopsy would surely agree that their first was a difficult, brutalizing experience. During the week after I had made this passage, I wondered about the wisdom of using the autopsy to introduce neophyte physicians to disease and death. Did the autopsy profoundly shake some students? Did it cause harm? Did it help foster denial or encourage the warrior mentality that many physicians are said to adopt? Did it drive people away from certain branches of medicine toward others where death occurred rarely?

One October evening I invited a few friends to dinner to explore reactions to attending an autopsy. After a few glasses of burgundy, tongues loosened and feelings flowed. The key themes that night were disgust and sadness. Bonnie spoke most forcefully.

"It was horrible, a revolting experience. When they opened his stomach and I could see the food, I almost vomited. The resident made stupid, immature jokes the whole time. He showed absolutely no respect for the body. I shall never attend another autopsy."

Steven picked up on the issue of respect. "Isn't it peculiar," he said. "As a dying patient that man was probably accorded great respect. Everything changed when he was laid out on the autopsy table. Why is that?"

"I don't think that the dissection, however brutal it may be, is in itself a disrespectful act," argued Dick. "It was the resident's attitude that really bothered Bonnie. But, Bonnie, look at it from his perspective. He's a young guy who is new to his bizarre job. I mean, this guy carves up people for a living. His bad jokes are to give him some distance, some breathing space. Maybe it's the only way that he can deal with it."

"That makes sense," said Bonnie. "But I don't agree with you about the dissection. Even conducted by the most gentle, sensitive pathologist, I would find the autopsy brutal and disgusting. It strikes me as an archaic, primitive rite. It is like a ritualistic punishment; the doctors exorcise their sense of failure by killing the already dead patient who refused to get well. I wonder whether it really still has scientific value."

"The organ review bothered me more than the autopsy itself," mused Steven. "It made me sad to see my corpse's organs strewn on steel strays in one room while his empty shell lay in another. To me the body has a unity that the organ review violates. I know that it sounds odd, but I think the pathologist should act more like a doctor. Doctors consult at the patient's bedside. Why can't pathologists review the organ analysis at the patient's table?"

"I think that we are telling each other a lot about our feelings toward death," said Dick. "We can't stop thinking of the body as a living thing. But, in a sense, a corpse is less important than a living insect. It is dead. Period. Like relatives, we are having trouble separating from the newly dead patient."

"Wouldn't it be much easier," I reflected, "if as a person died, he literally faded away? At the moment of death the body should just disappear. It is so cruel that a man dies but his body lingers on, not knowing what to do with itself, crying out for attention."

"Carry that a step further, Phil," urged Steven. "Wouldn't the world be happier if when a person died our memory of him faded as well? In minutes or hours all traces would be gone. There would be no pain. Of course, there would be no loving memories either. I think we just have to accept the reality of the dead body and learn to deal with it as fast as we can. Otherwise, we are heading into a lot of pain."

Bill, who had been quietly nursing an oversize can of beer, raised his head. "Speaking of the avoidance of pain, is there another lager in the fridge?" Thankful that the mood was broken, we turned to the latest class gossip, a much easier topic. The sigh of relief was almost audible.

About a week later another classmate and I decided to give the subject of death and autopsies one more go-round. We chose to hold our symposium at a sleazy place called the Anchor Bar, a haunt not frequently graced by medical students. Our original plans were rapidly altered. We had stumbled onto a golden opportunity to observe "future patients." For an hour we eavesdropped on several old rummies as they argued with the bartender, harassed the waitress, and lied mightily to each other.

Coincidentally, the most amazing tale involved medicine. One old guy who could barely stand was describing a fantastic machine that had the power to cure impotence. The suffering male need only grasp the metal rod and it gave "instant results"! He said that he had acquired the machine from a clinic in Cleveland for one hundred fifty dollars. But, despite its great value, he was willing to sell it for twenty-five dollars!

Alcoholics! David and I wondered whether it was even

remotely possible for medical students, insulated for years in temperature-controlled libraries, hatcheries for the professions, to understand how to deal with patients who had spent the last decade wandering in alleys. It was possible to imagine treating their infections or setting their broken bones, but it was surely impossible to attempt to change their hopeless lives. As we drove home, we figured that in many big-city hospitals these men would constitute a significant percentage of the population. What were we getting ourselves into?

I returned to the morgue about a dozen times that semester. My readings in history of medicine had a lot to do with this; for me the autopsy table was a direct link to the great decades of the nineteenth century, when a few hundred physicians struggled successfully to provide medicine with a scientific foundation. Despite its ugly side, the autopsy was an intellectually romantic experience. It bridged the gap between art and science, hinting both of the ancient priests who read entrails and of the electron microscopist who diagnosed renal disease.

On my last visit to the morgue I attended a medicolegal autopsy. On the table lay a huge bearded man whose skull had been smashed into his brains. He had been found alone in a car that had rammed into a metal pole. State law required that the medical examiner perform the autopsy to decide whether to list the death as an accident, a suicide, or, perhaps, as foul play.

"The key here," said the professor who was doing the case, "is to look for inconsistencies. Did this man die on impact, or was he dead before the car hit the pole? Did he die minutes after or hours before the accident? Was he poisoned by someone who used his car to create a clever cover-up?" He turned to me. "How do you think this man died?"

"I'd guess the obvious. He died of a massive skull fracture."

"How do skull fractures kill?"

I paused. Was this the beginning of an endless series of rigged questions?

"Lots of ways. He could have bled to death. The impact could have destroyed the tissues that control his ability to breathe."

"Agreed. When did he die?"

"I don't understand."

"At what moment did his body die?"

"When his heart stopped beating." It was half answer, half question.

"So the babies who go on the heart pump for surgery are dead during the operation?"

"No. How about five minutes after the heart stops, except where the person is on a heart-lung machine."

"Better. What are you suggesting?"

"That a person dies when his brain dies, when the brain cells suffocate from lack of oxygen."

"Agreed. So how do you decide about someone like this guy who makes it to an emergency room and gets put on a respirator? His heart keeps beating, he stops bleeding, yet his brain is a mass of bone fragments and mush."

"He's dead."

"The heart is still beating."

"But, most of the brain is gone."

"Would you be willing to unplug his respirator and pronounce him dead?"

"Yes."

"That would be a big mistake. If you ever get involved in such a situation, and you will, pronounce him dead first, then unplug the machine. That way there is no way that

anyone can argue that the damn respirator had anything to
do with your decision. It avoids allegations of manslaugh-
ter. That's how we handle organ harvests for transplanta-
tion."

That evening I strolled through the sunset over East
Rock Park and thought about how to decide if someone was
dead or not. Suddenly, this simple question seemed very
difficult. I recalled a story that a now retired physician had
told me about his internship in Indianapolis. One night he
rode an ambulance to the scene of an accident. A crowd of
several dozen people tightly circled a man sprawled motionless in an intersection. Here he had landed after being
struck and thrown by a speeding car. As he bent over the
man, it was at once obvious from the crazy angle at which
his right knee was pitched that the leg was badly broken.
My friend turned to the ambulance driver, who doubled as
a medic, and acutely aware of the crowd, spoke in his most
authoritative voice.

"Pete, get me a Thomas splint."

The assistant looked curiously at my friend for a moment, glanced at the crowd, and bent low to whisper his
reply.

"Doc, that guy's dead, ain't he?"

My friend looked again at the crushed skull in the pool of
blood, felt for a pulse, and nodded.

"Yes, Pete. Forget about the splint."

"You gotta use common sense in this business, Doc."

"You're right, Pete," said my friend.

With its unavoidable emphasis on death and its implicit
message that it was identifying the enemies who would
repeatedly challenge and defeat my clinical skills, the
pathology course dramatically influenced me. The sheer
immensity of the subject matter was awesome. The pathology text that I read had 1595 pages, and each 10¼-inch

by 7-inch page had two columns of 56 lines averaging more than six words per line. The index was 48 pages long with about 5000 separate entries! While studying two other major courses, we were expected to learn pathology in four months. Clearly, this was not humanly possible. How could I or others ever learn enough to become good physicians? But, however arduous, the study of pathology made the enemy real. The reward for long hours at the microscope, in the morgue, or propped up in front of a text was that disease became palpable. And, if you could touch it, you could struggle with it and, perhaps, defeat it.

Chapter 4

HISTORIES AND PHYSICALS

At Yale the great transition from lecture hall and laboratory to the hospital wards occurs during the fourth semester. Symbolically, there was a dramatic change in the geography of our education as well as in its subject matter. In December of our second year, the class breathed an audible sigh of relief and said good-bye to the overheated anatomy lecture room and the black-walled, coffinlike pathology auditorium. We would now perch on the ancient wooden seats in the upper reaches of Fitkin Amphitheater, located in the very heart of the Yale New Haven Hospital. Finally, we were crossing the street; the pillars of the Sterling Hall of Medicine were at our backs and the red brick of the old Winchester Building was in our eyes. From January to April we would spend several hours a day in the deep, dimly lit amphitheater, struggling to grasp the first secrets of *clinical* medicine that the initiates were finally willing to reveal.

The pedagogical center of this new semester was a supercourse called Introduction to Clinical Medicine, which was actually an amalgam of four courses: laboratory medicine, radiology, pathophysiology, and physical diagnosis. The lectures on laboratory medicine promised to be fairly straightforward. We would be taught how various diagnostic tests provide answers to questions asked by clinicians working on the wards. Beginning with routine studies such as the CBC (complete blood count) and the UA (urine analysis), the people in lab medicine promised to lead us to ever more esoteric tests, such as those used to confirm the diagnoses of collagen vascular diseases and other exotica. It was typical spoon feeding, and we would be comfortable with it.

From the start "baby radiology" promised to be a fun course. It met during the noon hour, when normal humans were relaxing over a sandwich. To make up for this cruelty, the instructor, a youngish, quick-witted woman who favored blue jeans, promised to turn it into a quiz game. We would play "guess the finding on the film." Like everything else in medicine one learned "rads" by studying thousands of cases. This was merely a beginning.

Pathophysiology used a seminar format to teach us how diseases accomplished their deadly work. We would be meeting three times a week for about two hours a session. At each meeting a different physician would lead us through the assigned clinical case studies. These cases would summarize the physical findings and laboratory test results of a "real" patient. It was our job to reach diagnostic conclusions and consider therapeutic alternatives. Thus, our first patients were imaginary beings, whom we had to reconstruct from the printed page. This, however, did not dampen our enthusiasm; at least we had finally begun to talk about people. I could sense the excitement in my classmates.

The most enticing course was physical diagnosis. This was a complicated enterprise that began simply as a lecture series but evolved rapidly. Yet again, the class was divided into groups of four. Each group would be meeting one or two evenings a week so that we could inspect each other with our shiny new stethoscopes, reflex hammers, and ophthalmoscopes. After using each other to try to learn one aspect of the physical exam (for example, percussion and auscultation of the lungs), we would meet with our "pre-clerkship" tutor, a doctor who had volunteered to observe and correct our inevitably sorry efforts. After a few weeks we would gradually shift from poking classmates to examining real patients, still under the watchful eye of a physician. At some point in the spring we would solo, performing alone our very first physical examinations on strangers, an exciting and frightening thought.

The lectures in the physical diagnosis course were given by Dr. Pierre Simon, a controversial theoretician who was struggling to "modernize" the art of clinical judgment. He had masterminded the format for the fourth semester, and he would be controlling our lives for the next three months. Simon, who specialized in criticizing the methods of clinical investigation, the major intellectual enterprise of academic physicians, was frequently at the center of debates in leading journals. During our months with him the controversy involved the validity of a gigantic study of the risks associated with using the birth control pill, probably the most widely used drug in the world. He had a curious and complicated reputation, and everyone was eager to hear him lecture.

We did not have long to wait. On the first day of our new semester Dr. Simon lectured for nearly three hours. A garrulous and intellectually sophisticated man, he was easily the most "verbal" lecturer we had in medical school. It was also obvious within minutes that he was clever, charming, and an unrepentant egotist. At the start he announced that he would learn all our names, a feat never even considered by our other professors. He then proceeded to delight us by already knowing the names of most students who asked questions.

After some preliminary banter, Simon began speaking with the intensity of an evangelist. Sweat glistened on his brow as he made his pitch to convert us. Peppering his lecture, which might have been titled "The Art of Knowing

Patients," with anecdotes, he held us spellbound. I was unsure as to what manner of disciples he would have us be, but the wild applause that he drew at the end of the day confirmed my suspicion that he was having a big effect.

Although I knew that the class was eager to begin clinical training and that this day had a special symbolic value, I was a little surprised at the rave reviews that Dr. Simon drew. He could be a bit condescending and seemed to enjoy the intellectual put-down. For example, when he was discussing the first moments in which a doctor and a patient, two strangers thrown into a very curious situation, interact, a student interrupted to ask what title we should use when we introduce ourselves. Visibly reddening, he seized the occasion to poke fun at people who worried about whether medical students should call themselves "doctor," dismissing this debate as "ethical masturbation." The students roared with laughter. Given that this had been a major subject for discussion among my classmates and that a substantial number had stated that it was wrong for students to hold themselves out as doctor, I was surprised by the storm of laughter. Were people's concerns so easily extinguished?

With the start of the fourth semester our workload seemed to double overnight. The Introduction to Clinical Medicine (ICM) course included twenty-eight hours of lecture time each week. Besides attending a reasonable number of these, we had to prepare for our pathophysiology seminars. In addition, we had to learn to take histories from patients and to perform physical examinations. This burden inevitably rekindled the pre-med anxieties (now part of the folklore of undergraduate life in America) from which many of the overachievers had suffered in college.

The most insecure and competitive people were the most vulnerable. During the first week of ICM I chanced to meet Anne and Allen, two of the more driven people in my class, having coffee. During our first year their competitive urges, which at times reached psychotic proportions, had made them infamous. Ironically, I now found them complaining that their classmates were too competitive. Trying to switch to a more palatable topic, I asked what they thought of the new course material. Anne started wailing.

"I can't keep up. No matter how much I work I fall further behind. I am sinking to the bottom of the class."

"Anne," I replied, "there's no class rank here. Relax. A minute ago you were criticizing people for being too competitive. But you just made a super-competitive statement. What gives?"

"You don't understand. People force us to do things we don't want to do."

I could feel the tremble in her voice and see the glaze falling over her eyes. Although she may have been asking for help, I was not up to the task. I beat a hasty retreat.

For the first two weeks of the new semester Dr. Simon remained the focus of our attention. One Friday he amazed us by conducting what he promised would be the "perfect" patient interview. Then, with a wave of his hand, he ushered in a middle-aged man who was sitting in a wheelchair. Acting like a magician about to perform the black arts, Dr. Simon first asked the man to confirm that they had not met until a few minutes earlier. Beginning with the classic question, What brought you to the hospital? during the next hour Simon probed every corner of the man's life. At the end of that time we knew an astounding amount about this man. Besides the obvious facts, that he was hospitalized with kidney stones and that he had undergone an appendectomy twenty years ago, we learned what kind of health insurance he carried, what kind of chemicals he was exposed to at work, and how often he made love with his wife.

We left the amphitheater convinced that Simon had kept his promise. Not only did he show us how much data one can elicit from a moderately cooperative patient, he proved that it was possible to include intimate and difficult questions about topics like sexuality as part of the routine history. Surely, if he could get a patient to respond before an audience, we could manage in a more private encounter. Finally, when he explained why he had asked many questions that had appeared irrelevant, he did much to reshape our understanding of why topics like social history and family history are important. Indeed, to Simon these questions were often the most crucial. By the end of the semester he had convinced us of the importance of psychosomatic problems in American culture.

As the weeks passed, I became enchanted with Simon's clinical prowess. He was, unquestionably, a brilliant physician, but there was a curious side to his personality that I never understood. He seemed to be obsessed with talking about taboo topics. When he wished to discuss a common disease, his most frequent choice was "pruritus ani"—in lay terms, an itchy anus. The first two or three times this topic earned a chuckle from the crowd. Yet, he sometimes persisted after the humor had worn thin. Like some of his colleagues, he also occasionally joked about sexual function, and even if the joke was bad, his leering grin drew laughter. I have wondered what heuristic value he saw in this material.

On the second Monday of the semester our physical diagnosis group met for the first time with our preclinical tutor, a young pediatrician named Carl Pelton. He was a chubby, bearded man who immediately put us at ease. Our first lesson was to master a very basic task: how to take a blood pressure. But no task is too easy for the beginner. When I started to put the cuff on my partner's arm, I realized that I had no idea how to wrap it so that the Velcro tape guaranteed a snug fit. Although I already had seen this done dozens of times, I had never really paid attention. The conclusion was painfully obvious: I had a lot to learn.

Later that day there was a disturbing finish to our pathophysiology seminar. Dr. Bergson, a famous lung specialist, had led an excellent discussion of the epidemiology and treatment of bacterial pneumonia. At the end of the session he surprised us with an invitation to visit a patient whom he was caring for in the intensive care unit. She was dying of a fulminant pneumonia that he suspected was Legionnaire's disease. Thinking that all invitations were orders, we marched after him to the ICU. The old woman lay there, ashen and comatose. In addition to pneumonia, she was in congestive heart failure, and her tissues bloated with water. Dr. Bergson pulled up the sheet and pressed his thumbs into her ankles. They left deep prints, as though he had pressed clay. So this was *pitting edema*. I winced as he pinched the skin of her forehead to show that she did not withdraw from the pain. After calmly reading the latest laboratory reports, he turned away from her to tell us that she would die in a day or two.

Despite her comatose state, our visit seemed to me to be an inexcusable invasion of privacy, both hers and that of the other patients in the ICU. Only a few feet separated the dozen of us from worried relatives at other beds. Yet we were bubbling over with clinical questions and gave no hint of sympathy. Still no one elsewhere in the ICU gave a sign of displeasure. I held my tongue and wondered if I was overreacting.

Unlike prior semesters when the workload eventually became routine, the class never seemed to develop a rhythm for the fourth term. Our ship had entered a squall. The workload, especially the pathophysiology case studies, became steadily more demanding. To prepare adequately for the three weekly sessions, one had to set aside about five hours on Monday, Tuesday, and Thursday evenings. There was just no time for the mountains of other material.

Everyone felt overwhelmed. Naturally, there was a dramatic rise in the frequency of parties. Hardly a weekend slipped by without some medical student offering his or her apartment for the supreme sacrifice. As the workload grew, the parties became steadily more atavistic. The evening did not start much before ten, but by midnight virtually no one in the crowd could pass a blood alcohol test. As they pulled long swallows of Jack Daniels, med students gravely speculated on the risks and benefits of liver disease. Four of my classmates had somehow managed to rent a palatial home from a faculty member who was spending two years abroad. This "fraternity house," also known as the "Animal House," was the site of the most successful parties. Their wine always carried the gift of forgetting. On not a few Saturday nights I heard some brilliant critiques of medical education, but the smoke and bourbon precluded solid neuronal connections.

One could make some really interesting observations at these parties. One time I realized that I had only seen my friends assembled for two reasons: to attend lectures and to engage in drunken revelries. It was also at parties that the very curious relationship between the men and women in the class was most apparent. The men, normally quite friendly during the week, kept their distance at a party. There seemed to be an incest taboo that prohibited sexual encounters (with a few infamous exceptions) between classmates. The males focused their attention almost exclusively on the nurses and women students from the school of public health who inevitably made the scene.

The evenings when my "physical diagnosis group" met to practice examining each other were among the most memorable in medical school. The four of us usually met around nine o'clock at somebody's apartment, armed with a six pack of Foster's, an excellent Australian beer, and our new instruments. Given that we did not yet have the slightest idea about how to examine people, these sessions were often ludicrous. One night our task was to practice listening to breath sounds. The instruction book suggested that we use magic markers to sketch the lung fields on each other. Without really thinking about it, we gravely followed this advice. My back and chest were soon crisscrossed with red lines, drawn painstakingly by a classmate in an effort to outline my lungs and liver. As the evening progressed and the lager diminished, we pondered the mysteries of bronchophony, egophony, and whispered pectoriloquy (words used to describe the quality of sounds heard through the stethoscope when the patient has various lung problems). Fortunately, at the end of these sessions we didn't care that we didn't know. We still had faith in the future.

The most difficult of our physical diagnosis sessions occurred one February afternoon when Dr. Pelton taught us how to do a rectal exam. Neither the privacy of the examining room, our serious purpose, nor the close alliance that the four of us had formed were enough to counteract our anxieties. We were about to shatter the glass of social convention. It was one thing to put a stethoscope on a friend's chest; it was quite another matter to stick a gloved and jellied finger up his rectum. Dr. Pelton tried to joke us into relaxing.

"OK. Who wants to be felt up first?"

There was a long silence. One of my partners mumbled something about having once had an "unpleasant experience." I decided to be the guinea pig. But there was method in my madness. Dr. Pelton would demonstrate on me; that, I reasoned, was less dangerous than submitting to the probing index fingers of any of my classmates. I quickly dropped my drawers, clambered onto the table, assumed the fetal position and tried to relax. Donning a glove, Dr. Pelton first instructed us on the critical importance of lubrication and helping the patient to relax. Instructing me to breathe deeply through my mouth, he then talked his way through the thirty-second exam. I can't claim that it is pleasant to have your prostate palpated, but it certainly was not as uncomfortable as I anticipated. "Besides," I thought as his finger slid out, "for me it's over. Now they have to go through it."

Perhaps the only thing as uncomfortable as submitting to a rectal exam by a friend is the embarrassment of being the examiner. Suddenly, a good friend with whom you have passed countless hours trying to master physiology is curled up naked before you on a cold, plastic examining table while you are inspecting his anus and preparing to shove a finger into his rectum. This is not an everyday test of friendship. It was my lot to examine Neal. Try as I might to locate his prostate (traditionally described as feeling like the bulb of one's nose), I could not. The only object I could identify was a large, well-formed stool, a finding which I dutifully reported to the laughing instructor. I am struck by how clearly I remember this half hour. These are the kinds of experiences that made medicine the curious fraternity that it is.

One snowy Thursday afternoon late in grim February, Dr. Simon gave his last lecture on the art of dealing with patients. It was one of those special moments when a rapt audience wholeheartedly hands itself over to the teacher. Simon had obviously enjoyed lecturing to us, and he waxed nostalgic in his farewell. He made old memories of his early years in medicine take life and parade before us.

Remembering how tough it is to be a beginner, he urged us never to forget that no matter how hard you have to work or how little sleep you get, the rewards were worth the sacrifice.

"Medicine," he said, "offers a front row seat on life. For the rest of your days people will bare their souls to you. If you retain the ability to savor this privilege you will all die rich."

Four days after Dr. Simon's last lecture, I took my first history from a patient. The physical diagnosis course required that we interview three patients and perform two complete physical examinations before the end of April. No one could argue that these experiences conferred competence, but they might assuage our feelings of terror when we anticipated starting on the wards in July. The patients upon whom we would practice taking histories were procured for us by our fourth-year tutors (there were so many different tutors in the physical diagnosis course that I never learned their titles). They were senior medical students who had virtually finished medical school. Only two years ahead of me, they spoke a language that I could not yet understand. They seemed wonderfully at ease in the hospital and had mysterious ways of producing patients for our benefit. My fourth-year tutor, a woman named Margery, had called me earlier in the week to say that a patient named Frank Bates would be expecting me on Monday evening at eight.

I spent late Monday afternoon pacing my attic apartment like an actor trying to memorize his lines. Although I had read about the proper method of conducting a history and had watched Dr. Simon in action, now that the moment was at hand there seemed to be hundreds of questions to ask, most of which I could not possibly remember. Realizing that I would accomplish little by cramming random questions between my ears, I concentrated on reviewing the essential topics.

There are six parts to the patient history: the chief complaint, history of present illness, past medical history, review of systems, family history, and social history. The patient's chief complaint is elicited with the classic opening line: What brings you to the hospital? The history of present illness is the most important element of the interview. The goal is to obtain a detailed description of the patient's problems. The physician must act like a detective. No point is too trivial for consideration, contradictory elements of the story must be explained, and diagnostic clues should be pursued with direct questions. Many doctors argue, rightly I think, that 90 percent of all diagnoses are made during the "history."

The past medical history encompasses other medical problems that the patient has faced but that are not clearly related to the current illness: childhood illnesses (measles, mumps, chicken pox?), prior hospitalizations, and all the surgical procedures undergone. It also includes a woman's pregnancy history. Besides giving the interviewer an impression of a patient's overall health, the past medical history can narrow the diagnosis. For example, if a person has undergone gallbladder removal, then the pain in the right upper quadrant is not due to cholecystitis.

The review of systems, which often is not given the attention it merits, helps the physician check for other *subclinical* problems patients might dismiss as trivial or unrelated to their main concern, but might be relevant and crucial. The ROS is used to scan quickly all organ systems (vision, hearing, endocrine, respiratory, gastrointestinal, and so on) for clues. One could ask several hundred questions during the ROS, but, realistically, one asks only a couple dozen broad questions to ensure that nothing obvious is overlooked and to force the patient to think about his or her body. The ROS questions are probably the most bewildering to the patient. There the patient sits in a hospital bed waiting to undergo cardiac catheterization in the morning and some medical student attacks with a machine gun fire of weird questions.

"Have you ever coughed up bright red blood?"

"No."

"Have you ever seen bright red blood in your bowel movements?"

"No."

"Have you ever urinated blood?"

"No."

Generally, the reaction to this inquisition comes in one of two ways. Either the patient says no to every question and the student quickly moves on, or the patient dutifully dredges up at least one problem in every organ system for the doctor to consider. Usually these are real but trivial complaints, which the examiner politely considers as rapidly as medical decorum permits.

The family history helps the doctor to identify "risk factors" for a particular disease. Given that there may be a biological predisposition to most illness and that genes are a critical factor in many diseases that people do not always think of as familial (cancer, hypertension, diabetes), the family history can be very informative. The complaint of chest pain in a thirty-year-old man changes dramatically when he tells you that his father died of an MI (myocardial infarction) at 47 and his brother had one when he was thirty-three.

The social history gives the doctor a picture of the overall state of a patient's life. Is he employed or on welfare? Is she married or recently widowed? Is he a long-time resident of the community or a newcomer? How much alcohol does she drink? How much does he smoke? Has she recently traveled outside the country? How much schooling did he receive? A thumbnail sketch of a patient's life may provide diagnostic clues, but it is especially valuable in giving the doctor an idea of the patient's ability to cope with his problems. For example, a widowed man or woman may be a lot more depressed than he or she admits and may need more emotional support than someone with a spouse.

Having pondered and paced away the afternoon, I fixed a quick dinner, slipped into a clean shirt, put on a tie, and donned my white coat. Remembering the fried onions, I stopped to brush my teeth. Somehow, while standing at the sink, I drifted into a fantasy. When I returned to reality a moment later, I realized that the mirror had seduced me. On this, my first official visit to meet a patient, the mirror had envied my white coat. For a moment I had been "Phil Reilly, young doctor," as omnipotent and caring as all those television physicians. I could only marvel at my capacity for foolishness.

The interview, miraculously, went quite well. Frank Bates, it turned out, was a delightful fifty-five-year-old man who had undergone a "triple" six days ago. The cardiothoracic surgeons had cracked his chest, pried the ribs back, and sewn pieces of a leg vein into the arteries that the heart used to nourish itself. They had done the operation because he was so incapacitated by ischemic heart disease that he could not walk from one room to another without getting bad chest pain. A cardiac catheterization had shown that his coronary arteries were clogged, as drain pipes after an autumn rain.

Mr. Bates, a widower without children, appreciated the break in the boring recovery routine. Fortunately, I remembered enough questions so that there were no long, embarrassing silences. By the end of an hour I really had learned a great deal about him. When he told me the history of his severe chest pain, a problem that had gotten much worse over the last three years, he spoke intensely; tears were in his eyes as he confided that he had not expected to see another summer.

Thanks to Mr. Bates I shall always remember that the

doctor and the patient see the business of history taking from dramatically different perspectives. History taking is as routine for the doctor as processing a loan application is for a bank officer. But the patient facing those questions may be devastated by his or her illness. At the least the patient may have a cloying fear that the funny new discomforts (nicely sanitized as "symptoms") are the harbingers of death. Such anxiety may make providing the history a super-charged experience. Communication between doctor and patient may also be compromised by a host of other obstacles: differences in age, sex, race, religion, education, and upbringing to name a few. Even though our society has defined the sick role to encourage open communication, there are a host of problems that can stymie a good medical history. Furthermore, the time pressures on the doctor may preclude careful attention to these problems. One has no choice but to acknowledge the constraints and do the best one can.

During the second half of February most of our energies were focused on the pathophysiology seminars. Topics of immense importance slipped past us with frightening speed. In a single week we covered congenital heart disease, acid-base disorders, and thyroid dysfunction. I felt as though I were standing before a conveyor belt watching information move by. The more I worked the less I seemed to learn. Each evening the price for seriously studying one topic was to learn nothing about the other assignments. Each time I remembered that the next time I dealt with one of these subjects it would be due to the illness of a real person, I winced.

The professors did little to alleviate our anxieties. Unlike the nice folks in the basic sciences, the clinicians were quick to criticize our competence. Within two weeks I must have heard my pathophysiology seminar group indicted for stupidity at least six times. These put-downs were probably intended to make us work harder, but they had the opposite effect. Attendance began to drop off, people began to admit defeat, and a few opted to spend their afternoons at the gym.

On February 23 we started a new phase of our preclinical training. Yet another permutation of students to which I had been assigned drove to St. Mary's Hospital in Bridgeport to begin our preclerkship tutorial. Our tutor, Dr. Martin Leonhardt, a former chief of medicine, was a small, energetic, friendly man. We learned that for the next six Wednesday afternoons he had arranged for two senior residents to help us examine patients who had obvious abnormalities that could be detected on exam. "Physical findings rounds," as we called them, were the next logical step in our clinical training. For a month I had been listening to the hearts and lungs and poking the nooks and crannies of four healthy young men. We had no idea yet what rales (a change in breath sounds in pneumonia) sounded like, and I had never felt an abdominal mass. We were positively eager to see, hear, and touch persons with disease. At the time I did not pause to marvel at how effectively we had been socialized into the physician's role.

My teaching resident was a curly-headed, athletic guy named Brian. He was finishing his medical training but had decided to take a second residency in orthopedic surgery, a fact that blew my mind. Four more years of residency—of sleepless nights and low pay. "Did one train forever?" I wondered. Brian took us to the ICU to visit a fragile old lady with pneumonia in both lungs. After cranking up the bed, he gently tugged her forward so we could place our stethoscopes on her back. The noises were unmistakably different from "normal" breathing. Fine, wispy sounds as though fingers were rubbing hair marked each inspiration.

Finally, I had heard rales! The art of diagnosis was a shade less mysterious.

The following Wednesday we examined two patients who provided us with an unforgettable moment in clinical education. The first was an elderly, rotund lady with dry, paper-thin skin, scant eyebrows, and a huge "butterball" face. She had a slow pulse and a sleepy way about her. Without telling us the diagnosis, Brian next led the way to the second patient. She was a young, slender black woman with silky skin and bulging eyes. Although none of us had been able to diagnose the first woman's illness, even neophytes could recognize Graves' disease. The black woman had hyperthyroidism and the other patient had hypothyroidism. Seeing patients with polar examples of thyroid dysfunction gave life to hundreds of paragraphs in our texts. This was the afternoon that I realized that a physician learns best from patients, not books.

On the ride from Bridgeport back to New Haven our talk turned to our anxieties over examining patients. James, who was fascinated with how patients perceive doctors, was troubled that Brian had described the lady's face as a "butterball" while standing in front of her. He felt that this was insulting and threatened the rapport between her and the doctors. I agreed but countered that it was also insulting to a patient to step outside the room for the obvious purpose of talking over his or her case. There did not seem to be a way to resolve the dilemma.

Our fourth visit to St. Mary's marked our first attempt to do doctor's work. That afternoon we would each subject a patient to a partial physical exam. For the first time, no tutor would be at our side. It was a small beginning, but a beginning nevertheless. Before leaving for Bridgeport I bumped into James in the men's room. We jokingly jostled for the attention of the mirror, looking like a couple of high school sophomores getting ready for the first dance. "Are your nails clean?" kidded James, recalling Dr. Simon's ad nauseum advice on the virtues of cleanliness. He inadvertently reminded me that becoming a doctor involves a lot more than learning to diagnose and treat illness.

My patient was an ancient Puerto Rican lady with valvular heart disease. When I realized that she spoke no English I groaned. I only had thirty minutes in which to do the physical. I had never examined a woman before, and here I was resorting to sign language to explain that I wanted her to disrobe! To my great relief she understood my talking hands and unhesitatingly unbuttoned her blouse. I had often wondered whether I would feel embarrassed examining a naked woman. Perhaps because she was so removed from me by age and language, her shriveled breasts did not make me uncomfortable. Self-absorbed, I did not worry about what she was feeling. For the next twenty minutes I listened to her two heart murmurs in every way I could remember, hoping that I would not prove a complete fool when Dr. Leonhardt asked me to describe what I had heard. Fear of ignorance neutralized whatever hangups I brought to this first professional encounter with female nudity.

There was lively discussion that afternoon as Neal weaved his red VW through the madness of Interstate 95. Still utterly bewildered by clinical medicine, we were wondering what forces shape the metamorphosis of medical student into doctor. We agreed that the key force was experience. Like it or not one had to see patient after patient. Like it or not one had to hoard facts like a miser who stuffs money into mattresses. At the moment we were just learning the most obvious clinical signs (like bulging eyes in thyroid disease) that anyone could identify. In time one might become adept at noticing really subtle physical signs. Maybe after twenty years and ten thousand patients one would have developed a "sixth sense" for physical diagnosis. Perhaps someday one might sense the answer before even posing the diagnostic questions.

As our "field trips" to hospitals became more frequent, I began to speculate on a provocative but troubling new topic: nurses. I started observing how nurses interacted with patients and doctors. The data were confusing. Some nurses were extremely knowledgeable and really asserted themselves about patient management. A few others, especially the youngest women, seemed to behave like stowaways on "Love Boat." By the same token there were a few male residents who were just as flirtatious.

One question perplexed me: How much do nurses know? Some nurses, particularly those who work in the coronary or intensive care units, were obviously far more knowledgeable than I about selected aspects of medical science. I remember feeling hopelessly ignorant the first time I overheard some CCU nurses debating the drugs that an intern had chosen to regulate a patient's heart rate. Only later did I wonder whether their knowledge was empirical or whether they knew the mechanism by which the drug worked. I was in a double-bind; one part of me worried that they would know far more than did I, the other part feared that they would not know enough. Clearly, it would take a while before I could learn how best to work with them.

On the last day of February I visited the West Haven VA Hospital for the first time. On countless occasions during the past two years I had driven beneath its commanding presence on a bluff overlooking New Haven harbor, each time knowing that sooner or later it would engulf me. This was the beginning. A group of us had been permitted to visit the stroke unit on the sixth floor.

We simply were not prepared for the first patient. The doctor, a gaunt man with piercing eyes and an unsympathetic face, had warned us that this man had been devastated by a brain hemorrhage. A hand-lettered sign at the

foot of the bed told us that his name was Ivan Modanko. He
lay face up and motionless on clean white sheets in a sunny
room surrounded by medical students, but cut off from the
world by a compromised brain. Among other injuries, he
could no longer speak. As the resident began to demonstrate a cranial nerve exam, I noticed that Mr. Modanko's
right hand was wrapped in a large bulky bandage and that a
tracheostomy tube jutted from his throat. Mr. Modanko
could obviously hear. He obeyed the instructions to follow
the doctor's finger with his eyes, a simple test proving that
cranial nerves three, four, and six were intact. As the exam
progressed, the extent of our patient's injuries became
more apparent. He could wrinkle only one side of his
forehead, he could barely open his mouth, and could not
stick out his tongue. This meant that part of his fifth,
seventh, and twelfth cranial nerves were not working.

The roughest moment came when we watched the resident test his "gag," a brainstem reflex mediated by the
ninth and tenth nerves. He wedged a tongue depressor
deep into the man's throat and stroked his pharynx. Mr.
Modanko gagged violently. This loosened a lot of phlegm
that he could not spit up, so he started choking. He was
drowning in mucus! The resident paused for a horrible
moment, then efficiently suctioned the junk from the
tracheostomy tube. The faces of several students contorted
with pain, and two people left the room.

In the corridor the physician asked if we had any questions. One student asked why he had not tested some other
reflexes. Before we knew it the resident marched us back
into the room. He twirled a wisp of cotton from a Q-Tip and
touched it to the man's cornea, causing him to blink
rapidly. This meant that a special arc involving the fifth and
seventh nerves was intact.

Later our host explained how the neurological exam
could be used to map the devastation wrought by a stroke.
This patient had had a stroke that had wiped out part of his

brainstem as well as tracts of nerves running through that area (as though a bomb had wiped out all but two lanes of the George Washington Bridge). We had all read about CVAs (cerebrovascular accidents), but nobody had anticipated the reality of their devastation. As we were moving on, I asked, "Why is his right hand bandaged?"

"He tries to kill himself by pulling out his trach tube," said the resident.

For a fleeting instant I thought, "Maybe we should let him."

We next saw a man with very advanced Parkinson's disease. The physician asked him to walk down the hall so we could see his classic shuffling gait. Walking as though wearing lead shoes, he barely got his feet off the ground. His face a mass of smacking grimaces, he appeared to have no control over his lips. This irreversible side effect of his medicine is called tardive dyskinesia. His roommate was a man with bizarre spastic torticollis. His head was at right angles to his shoulders, and he could not raise it to gaze forward. But the doctor could lift it with two fingers! Last we examined a man with a bizarre case of dysphasia. When he spoke, he made sounds that seemed like an alien language, but which were utter nonsense. Oddly enough, he could speak English obscenities, but nothing else was comprehensible. His gestures clearly said that he was trying to figure out why a bunch of strangers had invaded his privacy. What supreme frustration! Here was a man whose brain presumably had normal thoughts, but he could not express them, either orally or in writing. The cells that were supposed to do those jobs were dead. When we finally left the VA hospital that afternoon, it seemed more menacing than ever.

March 2 was a milestone. I conducted my first complete history and physical examination. The patient, Roger Hardy, was suffering from severe psoriasis (a disease that

may cause huge expanses of the skin to grow red and scaly).
He was extremely talkative, and, despite my best efforts to
focus the interview, the history took nearly ninety minutes. At sixty-seven, he was a proud grandparent who had
lived his entire life in Connecticut. Other than psoriasis,
his medical history was relatively simple, but his life
history was fascinating. As I listened, I remembered Dr.
Simon's admonition that medicine offered a front row seat
on life. Mr. Hardy had left school at the age of nine to work
for his father in the family-operated cigar factory. They had
grown, cut, and cured the tobacco and hand-wrapped the
cigars. They had printed their own labels and had sold
their product from horse-drawn carts on street corners.
After his parents' death, the business had failed and Mr.
Hardy had sunk into alcoholism. He took great pride in
telling how he had eventually won an eleven-year battle
with that disease.

I had conducted the history alone, but Nan, my fourth-
year tutor, arrived to observe the physical exam. For no
good reason I became nervous. To make matters worse,
when Mr. Hardy disrobed I saw that his body glistened
with a thick oily film—part of his treatment. I silently
cursed my tutor. Covered with oil and ugly, scaly skin, Mr.
Hardy was not exactly an easy patient to examine. Why
could she not have found me a patient with a simple
pneumonia? Was this a subtle form of hazing? Starting with
the head I moved quickly through the physical, leaving out
a quarter of the required steps.

In my haste I became sloppy. When I leaned forward to
perform a funduscopic exam of my patient's eyes, I slipped
on an oily patch of floor and struck his forehead with my
ophthalmoscope. Both my new instrument, for which I had
paid one hundred dollars and still had no idea how to use,
and I were covered in oil. Through the film, I could not see
the eye's vessels, let alone the optic disc (a yellow-white

spot where the optic nerve enters the back of the eye). I remembered to listen to Mr. Hardy's breathing, but I omitted the tests for fremitus, petriloquy, and egophony (sound qualities that indicate unusual densities in lung tissue). I forgot to feel most of his pulses (one traditionally palpates five symmetric spots on the body: neck, arm, wrist, groin, and foot). All in all, it was a disaster. When Nan reviewed my performance she devastated me with a single request: a description of Mr. Hardy's skin. I could not believe my ignorance, I had examined a patient whose only medical problem was psoriasis and I could not accurately describe his skin lesions. I had barely looked at them. That night I crawled home with my tail between my legs.

One of the more unusual requirements of our course in pathophysiology was to be observed by a psychiatrist while interviewing a patient whom we had never before met and about whom we knew nothing. The idea was that the psychiatrist would make constructive comments about our interview style. One Friday afternoon in March we met with Dr. William Brennan, a chief resident who had volunteered to observe. He asked me to interview a woman named Claire while he and my three classmates listened. We found her reading a magazine; I introduced everyone, took a chair to the far side of her bed to separate myself from the rest of the invasion party, and began.

Feeling on the spot, I started with some "safe" questions. Claire told me that she was thirty-two, divorced, and the mother of two children, eight and ten years old. They lived with her boyfriend in a tiny village in Rhode Island. She had grown up happily in Hartford, the middle child in a big, noisy, supportive family.

About five minutes passed before Claire dropped the

bomb. Almost casually she told me that she had just learned that she had leukemia. How does one respond to such an announcement? Deep inside I felt a sense of horror, but I contained it and tried to continue nonchalantly. Although the pitch of my voice did not change, I knew that, almost against my will, I was now asking a different set of questions. I retreated into the role of the doctor, seeking clinical facts. For the next forty minutes I hugged the outline of the straight medical history, only occasionally asking more general questions. After I stopped, Dr. Brennan said a few words; then we bid Claire good-bye and trooped back to his office to dissect the interview.

I thought I had done a pretty good job, but the group had quite a few criticisms. They thought that I had talked too much, and that I had seemed uncomfortable when asking intimate questions. Ron noticed that I tended to preface my questions by saying, "If you don't mind me asking." James felt that I tried too hard to identify with the patient. For example, when she mentioned that she worked as a bartender, I had said "I've done that too." Dr. Brennan may have pointed out the worst flaw. He said that as soon as I had learned that the lady had leukemia, I had started emphasizing the positive in every possible way—a transparent therapeutic maneuver.

Our opinions about Claire differed radically. I felt that she was dealing well with her illness, but James and Ron felt that she was very depressed. Needless to say, an interview might be conducted differently depending on which opinion one held. As we broke up Dr. Brennan offered one excellent bit of advice. "Always ask the patient if he knows somebody with the same problem." This may be the easiest way to ascertain how familiar he is with his new disease. Talking about someone else also gives the patient a chance to distance himself momentarily from the disorder.

On my next trip to St. Mary's I made a special effort to apply the ideas Dr. Brennan had raised. Although our task there was still merely to elicit physical findings, I tried to listen carefully to what patients said about their illnesses. I was quickly rewarded. The first person I visited was an old woman with acromegaly. Her physicians "knew" that her growth problem (her hands and face were enlarging) was caused by a derangement of her pituitary gland, but she "knew" that all her problems started right after her husband had died four years earlier. Suffering from constant headaches, she steadfastly refused the surgery she needed. She was leery of doctors and frightened that she would die in surgery. Yet, she thought her personal physician was the "best in town," a man who "stood over all the other doctors." How often since then have I heard patients embrace this contradiction: They distrust every doctor but their own!

The visits to St. Mary's were interesting for other reasons as well. After each experience I could identify a few new facts that had been added to my slender library of medical knowledge. The progress, however slow, was visible and encouraging. On the same day that I met the lady with acromegaly, I also examined a patient with Dressler's syndrome, a condition that I had never before heard discussed. As he tried to help us listen to her "friction rub," our resident explained that two weeks after a heart attack some patients get a transient pericarditis (inflammation of the tissue that outlines the heart) and have sharp chest pain that lasts for a day or two. This must be scary, but it is not a second heart attack and it quickly resolves.

One of the more difficult days in medical students' lives is the day they attempt their first pelvic examination. Even under ideal circumstances the chance of a rewarding experience is remote. Whether they admit it or not, most students, teachers, and patients are shackled by the psychosexual taboos of the culture. From the start the pelvic exam is "different" from other parts of the routine physical, and a different approach is required. Since this is a nondangerous, brief, and crucially important investigation, it is really too bad that it is shrouded with problems.

In the old days medical students frequently learned to feel the female pelvic anatomy on anesthetized patients. After the patient was asleep (and without any concern for informed consent), the surgeon would call students to the operating table and instruct them on the insertion of a speculum and the examination of the cervix. Over the last decade, coincident with the dramatic increase in the number of women entering medicine, students have objected strenuously to learning pelvic examinations in this manner. Medical school officials have tried a number of alternatives, none particularly successful. The most common solutions have been to pay healthy volunteers to undergo repeated exams (at least one school hired prostitutes, perhaps thinking that these women might need pelvic exams). Another popular solution has been to have students practice on lifesized molded rubber dummies, an experience that inevitably generates a current of tasteless jokes. Of course, teaching students to examine dummies only delays the inevitable; sooner or later the flesh will be real.

As at many schools, there had been controversy at Yale about how to teach the pelvic examination. The plan seemed to vary each year. My year a group of private obstetricians who attended at the women's clinic agreed to ask their patients to permit medical students to perform a supervised pelvic exam. I was one of four students who would be taught by Dr. Heger, a bluff, middle-aged German man. First, he guided our examination of the model, a bizarre torso and thighs complete with vagina and plastic cervix. There were even several rubber uteruses, each with a different pathological problem, that could be placed in the dummy. Dr. Heger wisely put all his energy into teaching us to use a speculum so that we would not cause the patient pain. Over and over again each of us inserted it at an angle, gently rotated it, and slowly expanded the blades, confident that the plastic cervix would pop into view.

After that we sat and waited for his patients to arrive. Over the next hour two patients did show up, and he led two classmates through an uneventful exam. When my colleagues reported that their exams had gone smoothly, I started to relax. Indeed, when Dr. Heger took time to demonstrate various cervical smears under the microscope, I actually enjoyed myself. But the afternoon was rushing toward four o'clock, the hour when clinic ended, and "my" patient had not appeared. Finally, at three forty-five, Heger announced that he had to leave. He towed me down the corridor and handed me over to a surprised resident with orders to "let the student do a pelvic."

Things immediately began to go wrong. Two minutes later I was standing in a tiny cubicle with the resident and a nurse facing an obese seventy-year-old woman who had not seen a gynecologist in twenty-five years. The resident, obviously pressed for time, took a rapid history, learning that the woman had come because of intermittent vaginal bleeding. She was obviously terrified that she had cancer, but if he realized her fears, the doctor certainly did not acknowledge them.

We stepped out of the cell for a moment so she could "assume the position," as he put it. When we stepped back in she was up in stirrups with a sheet draped over her legs. The resident propelled me to the three-legged stool at the end of the table, tipped the light so it shone on her vagina, and handed me a speculum. I felt terrible. No one had asked her to approve an examination by a student. I knew that I should refuse to examine her, but my desire to learn overcame my ethical concerns and I kept silent. With the resident literally breathing down my neck, I tried to pretend that this was just another rubber dummy.

Even before I touched her with the speculum she was moaning and I was sweating. Every time I tried to insert this odd-looking instrument she inched away from me and started to cry. Finally I managed to insert it, but I could not find the cervix. After two or three horrible minutes that seemed like as many hours, I gladly relinquished the stool and the resident took over. He quickly located and swabbed the cervix and then did a rapid bi-manual exam (with one hand in the vagina and the other hand on the abdomen, the examiner tries to feel uterus and ovaries). After he had finished I mimicked his exam, feeling nothing but her soft, fat belly. As soon as possible I fled the scene, not wishing ever to see that doctor, nurse, or patient again.

By mid-March I was seeing patients quite regularly. Despite my good intentions, however, I usually was so concerned about mastering whatever specific task I had been assigned that I often forgot that I was dealing with other human beings. The physical finding was more important than the patient. Fortunately, a chance remark by a woman at St. Mary's pulled me back to reality. She was suffering from a form of leukemia that carried the fancy label *agnogenic myeloid metaplasia*. Dr. Leonhardt took us to examine her abdomen. Mrs. Sanford greeted us warmly, and for the next twenty minutes she patiently allowed each of us to poke her belly. Even for a beginner the finding was obvious. Her spleen had swollen to five or six times its normal size. The entire left side of her abdomen was filled by a huge, frisbeelike mass. She did not seem to mind our too obvious fascination with her dying body. As I was about to lay my hands on her, I was struck by her gentle answer to my perfunctory request for permission.

"May I examine you?"

"Yes. I let you touch me so that someday you can save somebody else's life."

Her face was at once solemn and loving; she appeared almost beatific. Clearly, at that moment she had a much deeper understanding of the journey that I was starting than I had of the one she was finishing. This gentle, good woman, how could I appreciate her enough?

The next day I met a physician whose attitude contrasted sharply with the dignified, humble ways of Mrs. Sanford. A senior resident in ophthalmology, he was to lecture about the eye exam. We did not learn much about eyes that afternoon, but we did get a good look at an arrogant physician. Dr. Ellis spent an hour gloating about how much insurance companies pay for cataract operations ("$935 for a thirty-minute job"), his favorite sports car (Porsche Targa), and the virtues of owning stock in certain small pharmaceutical companies. His behavior was so blatant that at first I thought he was joking, but gradually I realized that this was no caricature. Concluding his fiscal musings, Ellis spent a few minutes trying to scare us about the upcoming national board examination. He posed a series of "simple" questions ("Name all the foramina through which the cranial nerves pass"), and he snorted with disgust when we could not answer. Fortunately, by this time I knew he was a jerk and refused to feel intimidated.

One of the more curious aspects of medical education is the use of mnemonics. The degree to which many medical students rely on mental shorthand suggests the intellectual depths to which we are reduced by mountains of facts. At first I hated mnemonics and looked down my nose at people who relied on them. Anatomy was the course in which this practice was most rampant. The most famous, which every medical student learns, orders the twelve cranial nerves (Olfactory, Optic, Oculomotor, Trochlear, Trigeminal, Abducens, Facial, Auditory, Glossophary- ngeal, Vagus, Accessory, and Hypoglossal). One version goes: "On Old Olympus Tiny Top A Finn And German Viewed A Hop." Needless to say, over the years medical students have devoted much creative energy to mnemon- ics. Not a few have invented scatological masterpieces. During my first months visiting the wards, it surprised me that even residents sometimes relied on mnemonics. For example, a neurology resident told me to remember the nine major causes of coma with the mnemonic: AEIOU TIPS. The vowels stand for: Alcohol, Encephalopathy, Insulin, Opiates, and Uremia. TIPS stands for: Trauma, Infections, Psychiatry, and Stroke.

By late March several of my classmates had metamor- phosed into mnemonic freaks. Eventually, I succumbed to the temptation. Searching for a word with which to re- member the five major causes of metabolic acidosis, I came up with MEDUSA. This stands for Methanol poisoning, Ethylene glycol poisoning, Diabetes, Uremia, and SAlicy- late poisoning. Mnemonic freaks may be identified by the three-by-five index cards they carry. MEDUSA might look like this:

M   ethanol poisoning
E   thylene glycol poisoning
D   iabetes
U   remia
S   alicylate poisoning or
A   spirin poisoning

Once when walking down a hospital corridor I found an index card with the mnemonic asserting that the "causes of high levels of calcium" could be reduced to the phrase: CHIMPS BAG. According to the inventor, C stood for calcium, H for hyperthyroidism, I for intoxication, M for milk-alkali syndrome, P for piss (as a reminder that some diuretics could cause hypercalcemia), S for sarcoidosis, B for berylliosis (metal poisoning), A for Addison's disease, and G for some indecipherable term. I wonder if more time was spent creating these mental shortcuts than was saved by using them.

Early in April the fourth semester ground to a halt. At the last possible minute, our class started working on the "second-year show." About eighty people (a few classmates were just too anxious about school to participate very much) put away their stethoscopes, closed their books, and skipped their pathophysiology seminars. Almost everyone pitched in to create, choreograph, and rehearse twenty skits, written with an eye to getting laughs and, in a few cases, getting even. Well-hidden talents blossomed. Some of the skits were multimedia events: One classmate (now a leading young cancer researcher) produced a "feature film" complete with synchronous sound; another borrowed the tunes from *Fiddler on the Roof* to create a spoof that was worthy of Broadway.

Egos blossomed even faster than talents. There was no shortage of actors who wanted to star in every skit. All the peacocks were spreading their feathers, and some were getting ruffled. Casting the show, titled *The Heartbreak of Satyriasis*, turned out to be a superb way to figure out which of our classmates was most competitive.

Heartbreak was a stupendous success. Our class played to a sell-out crowd in Sterling Auditorium. The skits flowed smoothly, leaving no facet of medical education unexamined or unsatirized. The physicians who had often marveled at our ignorance of anatomy were fondly remembered in "Samurai Surgeon." The Department of Pharmacology, a bunch of heavy hitters, were spoofed in "The Godfather," a skit portraying them as drug smugglers. One uninhibited classmate performed a solo skit as a television chef. Instead of describing the "nouvelle cuisine," he extolled the gustatory secrets in "bread and butter" *pericarditis*, nutmeg liver, and strawberry *hemangioma*. "Tasting" each specimen as he worked, the world's only culinary pathologist successfully nauseated the audience.

The second-year show marked the start and finish of my acting career. I starred in a commercial—a thirty-second monologue and slide show that imagined a day when antipsychotic medications were routinely dispensed by fast food restaurants. *Heartbreak* symbolically ended two years of anxiety and claustrophobia. The show's finale was a dance number superbly choreographed to a current rock hit. For an encore the entire class—one hundred people who had been stuffed into the same small lecture halls month after month—joined on stage and exuberantly repeated the dance number. We had come out of the closet.

My last official act of the fourth semester was to do a "complete" physical exam on a patient at St. Mary's hospital. It was a fiasco. I was assigned to examine a man with advanced "oat cell" cancer of the lung who was near death. He was semicomatose and uncooperative, so I spent the first few minutes wondering how I could move him about. Just as I had managed to roll him to one side, two doctors and a nurse armed with a thoracostomy tray marched in. Reflexively, I retreated. In an effort to drain his lung infection they were going to insert a chest tube. The plan was to numb the tissues and then stick a trocar (a polite word for a small spike) between his ribs. Despite the anesthetic, the man screamed and stuggled violently. The resident cut a vessel, and blood spurted all over the bed. Swearing mightily, the senior surgeon stepped in, quickly stopped the bleeding, and brutally maneuvered the trocar to make a hole. Next he put a gloved finger into the lung cavity to look for a collection of pus that had been sus-pected on x-ray. When he did not find the *empyema,* he quickly sewed the man up. Needless to say, after this experience the patient wanted nothing to do with me, and I was so troubled by the violence of this scene that I had no wish to trouble him further. I ended my fourth semester by lying to my instructor about the findings of a physical exam that I had not really performed.

The semester ended with a whimper. The last lectures had been weeks ago, and there were no final exams. April turned into May, and we just stopped. The next six weeks were devoted to studying for the national boards (a three-part exam given at the end of the second, fourth, and intern years, which medical students must pass to get licensed). After that there would be a three-week vacation, and then in July we would start our third year of medical school "on the wards."

Looking back, I think that the big lesson I learned that spring was not in pathophysiology, radiology, or physical diagnosis. What I learned (or started to learn) was how to communicate with patients. It was an extraordinarily rich period. Each visit to a patient was like reading an autobiog-raphy. Never before had I had such a sense for the diver-sity of human experience. There was Mr. Leonard, a man with renal cancer, who had run away at thirteen to join the Merchant Marines and who had never seen his parents again. There was Miss O'Connor, a ninety-nine-year-old woman who had grown up on a farm in Brooklyn, who, after being admitted to St. Mary's Hospital with hepatitis, wondered if she should cut back on her alcohol consump-tion! And there was Mr. Beadle, a ninety-three-year-old veteran of the Spanish-American War (he had been a drummer boy at San Juan Hill) who had been hospitalized with prostatitis. Each one of their stories was equal to the best of Tolstoy. Dr. Simon was right; medicine gave one a front row seat on life.

Chapter 5

FIRST MEDICINE

The six-week reading period allocated for preparation for part I of the national boards seemed interminable. Not having been formally examined by machine-graded tests during our three semesters of classroom study, many of us labored under a cloud of anxiety. Yet, try as we might, the monumental task of reviewing anatomy, biochemistry, cell biology, genetics, microbiology, pathology, pharmacology, and physiology defied completion. To me the task seemed almost absurd. Knowing that I could not keep the various steps of the urea cycle on my mind for more than twenty minutes, why should I study any biochemistry several weeks before a two-day, sixteen-hour examination? I passed a disproportionate amount of May and June worrying rather than studying. This was made especially easy by the glorious early days of summer.

As such days do, the examination days arrived. Our class once again reassembled to sit hunched over in crowded quarters and do battle with the first multiple-choice examination that we had seen in medical school. Blissfully, I have a nearly complete amnesia for the event. The list of questions was huge and the time to answer each so short that if one had any doubts, there was no choice but to guess and move on. After each of the four sessions into which this ordeal was divided, I and not a few of my colleagues became more convinced that this exam was easy to fail. The fact that we would have to wait several weeks for the results and that failure would result in the humiliation of being "pulled" from the hospital wards made the experience quite unpleasant.

My anxiety did not dissipate with the completion of the examination. Entry into the mysterious world of clinical medicine loomed ahead. After a brief vacation, during which I miserably failed to contain my fears about the unknown challenges that awaited me, I returned to face the beginning of my third year of medical school.

One of the few statements with which most physicians would agree is that the third year, the year on the wards, is the critical year in medical education. I would spend forty-five of the next fifty-two weeks rotating through six (presented in order) clerkships: obstetrics and gynecology, first medicine, psychiatry, surgery and surgical subspecialties, pediatrics, and second medicine. This experience was intended to provide us with exposure to most of clinical medicine and to help us choose the specialty in which we would train after graduation. Of course we could not gain exposure to every specialty in a single year. For example, there was no opportunity to study ophthalmology. This meant that the students who wished to become eye physicians had to make that choice (that is, apply for residencies) with no clinical experience. How could they make a career choice with so little information? Nevertheless, several of my more prescient classmates did choose ophthalmology.

My first clerkship, obstetrics and gynecology, was the stretch of the medical school marathon in which I stumbled badly. A number of factors contributed to my disastrous July and August, but the biggest factor was me. The first clerkship is difficult for a number of reasons. Students are not familiar with even the simplest aspect of the daily routine of hospital life. They must learn to function in an alien culture. The residents with whom and for whom they work have the significant burden of fulfilling genuine clinical duties for the first time. Residents *really* are responsible for patient care. In order to master their art, they may exclude students from all but the most peripheral involvement (usually, doing errands). Pleasant summer weather certainly does not encourage senior physicians to spend extra time in the hospital to teach neophytes. It is also vacation time when staffing may be tight. One consequence is that medical students may be pressed into chores for which the term *drudgery* would be a euphemism.

Perhaps because I was older than many medical students, the shock of realizing just how low on the rungs of the medical ladder (best described as a hole several feet below ground) I stood hit me hard. I spent the entire six weeks of my obstetrics and gynecology clerkship in a funk. Despite the extremely high quality of the obstetrics department, I felt that little attention was being devoted to teaching the new "ward clerks." My residents, themselves new to the task, were reluctant to let me deliver babies (I delivered only two during my three weeks on the obstetrics service). We were required to be "on call" in the hospital all night every third night, yet we were not permitted to do much and had no adequate place to sleep. On my first day on the gynecology rotation a resident described a patient with cancer of the vulva and then suggested I go to the library across the street and read about it. I recall that when I bumped into one of the few clinical professors I knew personally and he learned what I was studying, he started laughing. Cancer of the vulva, however worthy of study, is quite rare and hardly a topic on which a medical student should start. Of course, you have to begin somewhere.

To add injury to insult, one morning after an all-night vigil awaiting the birth of reluctant babies, I found that my car, parked on a deserted side street, had a window shattered with a brick. That was the last straw. Really unhappy, I broke some rules and fled to Cape Cod for the weekend to visit old friends (college classmates who were far more established than I). Fortunately, this breather helped me crawl through the rest of the clerkship.

Miraculously, with the end of the obstetrics clerkship, I pulled out of my funk. I was scheduled to spend the next six weeks on "first medicine," a clerkship famous for its teaching in a department that was filled with renowned physicians. Since roughly one-half of my class planned to compete for the top medical internships in the United States and because letters of recommendation were crucial, we regarded the two medical clerkships as the most critical part of our third year.

I was assigned to G3W, a general medical floor at the West Haven Veteran's Administration Hospital, affectionately known among generations of Yale students as the "VA Spa." Until my arrival that August morning I had only the vaguest impression of life at this sprawling 800-bed unit. The main building, an imposing ziggurat of red brick that had been finished in 1950, commanded a hill overlooking Interstate 95 as it swept down the coast to Manhattan. From the highway the hospital looks like an aging fortress. Inside its gates the world recedes and the place seems other-worldly; time moves at a different pace, reminiscent of the sanitorium described by Thomas Mann in *Magic Mountain*.

I liked the VA Spa immediately. No more parking on ghetto streets, no more bricks heaved through my car windows! Within minutes of my arrival a security guard had gotten me a parking sticker. Such treatment was unheard of at Yale. Being a few minutes early for rounds, I plopped down in the waiting lounge and reviewed the various handouts I had received. There would be two other medical students: Joseph Garola and Anthony Todman. I breathed a huge sigh of relief. Perhaps the greatest fear of a medical student is to be assigned to a ward team that includes a known turkey. If fellow students were super-competitive, super-obsequious, or super-dull, one's life could be utterly miserable.

Joseph was a hard-working type who was totally committed to becoming a doctor. A young, dark-haired Californian who always sported a smile, he was a bit ingenuous and a little too eager, but he was also friendly and fair. I knew we'd get along. Anthony was Mr. Cool. A quick-witted New Yorker who had graduated from Princeton, he favored unconventional clothes, longish hair, and a style that would insulate him from the "pre-med" image. He had an over-sized ego which craved attention, but he was also good humored and much too concerned with his image to be overtly competitive. Despite the fact that I could not match their drive or their intelligence, I felt easy. We would get along fine.

At about nine o'clock I climbed the cool green stairway up the five flights to find Joseph and Anthony and meet the chief resident. A few minutes later, as the three of us were sipping coffee in a small, austere conference room, he strode into our lives. Dr. Thomas Marshall—not an inch under six foot five, balding, and without the hint of a smile—reminded me instantly of a giant carnivorous bird, a distant cousin of the archaeopteryx, on the edge of extinction. We three little medical students would hardly make him a good meal.

From the first word he was all business. "Welcome to the VA. You are about to begin the most important six weeks of your life. Starting this morning you are a member of the medical team. I know you don't know squat, and I know you are scared. You should be. It's tough starting out at the bottom, but that is where everyone starts in medicine. You are here to work hard. This is not a part-time job. If you don't want to put out, you might just as well quit now because there is so much to learn it's frightening. All the residents and interns are willing to teach. But they have a lot to do, so teaching will be in fits and starts. One thing's for sure. They will be able to teach a lot more if you help them finish the daily chores as quickly as possible. Remember that." He paused and slowly fixed each of us with a piercing stare.

"Now I am not so far removed from med school that I have forgotten what it is like. Let me give you three pieces of advice. First, always keep your eyes and ears open. Sure, rounds can get mighty boring if they're not talking about your patient. But someday you will get a patient like the one that they are discussing while you daydream. Second, ask questions if you don't understand something. It's the only way to learn. But don't butt in, wait for the moment. Third, medicine is learned at night. We can't make you stay here all night when you're on call. But, late at night there's not many folks around. If a patient codes or there is an emergency admission, you will be able to get involved to a degree that just doesn't happen during the daytime. Any questions? No. Good. OK. Let's go join the team."

First medicine had begun.

The team consisted of two residents, two interns, and two subinterns (fourth-year students, each sharing half an intern's patient load). We found them just finishing rounds. After a flurry of introductions, the interns dispersed to work and the residents took us on a brief tour of the floor. John Caskey was the senior resident. Tall, muscular, and blond, he looked like a candidate for the US olympic swimming team. His laconic manner and quiet self-assurance set me at ease. Here was a man who knew what he was doing. Carol Fannin was the "JAR," the second-year resident. She had graceful manners and the most mellifluous Tennessee accent I had ever heard. I liked her instantly.

We began our tour at the far west end of the building in the coronary care unit (CCU). As we moved through the CCU, which had six single bedded rooms surrounding a nursing station, I felt terrified. Five years earlier I had visited the NASA Command Center in Texas. There seemed to be more fancy telemetry equipment crammed in this little CCU than in all of Houston. How was I ever going to learn all this? As I watched Carol and the head nurse consult a monitor and talk about *holtering* some patient, my heart sank. I had no idea what they were talking about. From the CCU we took the long walk back to "our" side (a different team covered the west ward) to the medical intensive care unit (MICU). The MICU was a large chilly room with eight beds separated by curtains. The nursing station formed a foyer separating the beds from the rest of the floor. Like the CCU this place was also laden with electronics; a TV console was suspended over every bed. This morning the pace was quite slow; four of the eight beds were empty and three of the patients looked relatively comfortable. But the patient in bed eight did not look good at all.

According to the sign taped over the bed, his name was Andrew Connally. He lay flat on his back, tangled in a maze of polyethylene tubing. At the foot of the bed was a pale green robot about the size of a dishwasher that sent wires to a white blanket covering him. This was a heating unit. At the head of the bed was a blue robot of about the same size. From the blue robot's side ran two plastic hoses that were joined to a tube in the man's mouth. Lettering on its side proclaimed that it was a Bear MA-2 respirator. Perhaps sensing my discomfort, John led us over to the bed.

"This man has severe COPD, chronic obstructive pulmonary disease. Before being hospitalized his breathing was so bad that he was restricted to sitting in a chair. He got a pneumonia last week and he had so little reserve that he was placed on a respirator almost immediately. We have him on all the right medicines, but as you can see he's not doing well. He's just barely responsive."

To prove his point John spoke loudly into the man's ear, asking him to open his eyes, but got no response.

"Let's take a minute to look over the console of a respirator," said John. The device appeared simple enough to operate. The console had about twenty separate dials and indicators arranged on a dashboard about two feet square, but only a few facts were important. Was the device assisting or controlling the patient's breathing effort? At what rate were "breaths" being delivered? At what volume? What mixture of oxygen had been chosen? Normal air is 21 percent oxygen, a little water vapor, some polluting gases, and mostly nitrogen. The average healthy adult male breathes about twelve times a minute, moving about five hundred cubic centimeters of air with each breath. This much I knew. At a glance I could see that each minute the patient was receiving eight breaths of 40 percent oxygen, each at a volume of five hundred cubic centimeters. John showed us we could look at a pressure gauge to tell if the patient was making any effort to breathe on his own. This man was not. I shuddered and we moved on.

The rest of the morning flashed by in a rapid series of tours and introductions. But by two o'clock we were free to learn the facts that were important to medical students. Where was the blood drawing cart? What were the phone numbers of the chemistry, bacteriology, and hematology labs? Where were the vending machines? How could one get into the x-ray file room late at night? The list was endless. That night at home I propped up my aching feet, popped open a beer and wondered what was in store for me. I soon found out.

The first week of my medical clerkship was one of the most extraordinary of my life. It was the week that I became *familiar* with death. For me, like many people in my generation, death's menace seemed remote and unreal. All but one of my grandparents had died before I was old enough to comprehend their passing. I had been two thousand miles away when my dear grandmother died. To this day I have never been to a funeral. The televised body counts that marked the progress of the Vietnam War had been too sanitized and unreal, too much like a movie, too far away to be believed. Once, before I went to medical school, while walking through the basement corridors of a big-city hospital, I had opened a back door and nearly stumbled over a corpse lying silently on a table in back of a giant black hearse. I had shrunk back in horror and hurried away.

It was Carol who unwittingly introduced me to death. After lunch on our first day she assigned each of the new students a patient to "pick up." We were to read the patient's chart and become responsible for helping the intern with his care. One by one she took each of us to meet our first patients. My patient was Mr. Webster. According to his chart Mr. Webster was a sixty-four-year-old black man who had been admitted ten days ago for a TURP, a transurethral resection of his prostate gland, the operation that keeps so many urologists smiling. His medical history was not remarkable, and he was just about ready to go home when, two days ago, he had had severe chest pain and had been transferred from a surgical to a medical floor. His EKGs were all normal and the chest pain had not recurred, so he would be watched for another day or two and then sent home.

Carol greeted Mr. Webster with a big smile. It was easy to see why she liked him. He had a white fringe of curly hair surrounding a brown dome, a white mustache, and a dignified air. Leaning forward slightly on a carved wooden cane, he sat on the edge of the bed in a red bathrobe. Carol explained my position in life and asked Mr. Webster if he would permit me to become involved in his care. "Sit down, sir," he said, "and I'll tell you everything you wish to know."

The next half-hour was delightful. I already knew most of Mr. Webster's medical history from the chart, so I concentrated on talking with him as one might chat with a friendly stranger on a tiresome bus ride. A lifelong resident of Connecticut, born and raised in Bridgeport, he had worked mostly as a security guard and had been chief of security at a small factory before his retirement two years ago. He retired early to tend to his wife, who had died of cancer six months ago. He had one son, a carpenter who lived with his family in Hartford. His son had been a great high school athlete, Mr. Webster told me, beaming with pride. He lived alone now and life was too quiet, but he liked his long walks in the park, where he often spent afternoons watching the children play. As I got up to leave, he thanked me for my visit, somehow making me feel as though I were his doctor. I assured him that we would visit again tomorrow.

Rounds began at eight o'clock in the morning. Nine of us gathered at the main nursing station to begin the long trek from room to room, hearing about changes in each patient's care and listening to the interns present the "new players"—patients who had been admitted during the night. We were about ten minutes into my first "rounds," walking down the corridor to the MICU, when Carol said to me, "Isn't it too bad about Mr. Webster?"

"What happened?"

"Oh, you haven't heard? He died last night. The nurse found him at six A.M. There was no code or anything. It was probably a pulmonary embolus, but we won't know until after the post this morning."

Our conversation stopped there as we started the round on the patients in the MICU. But I paid no attention. My first patient had died within hours after I met him. I simply could not believe it. Suddenly, a new duty loomed up. My job was to learn clinical medicine, and in this business your patients were your professors. Mr. Webster still had something to teach me; it was my job to attend his autopsy.

The morgue was a small, untidy, windowless room in the subbasement of the building. There were two autopsies in progress. My timing was perfect. Mr. Webster lay on the steel table with his chest and abdomen slit open. The incision ran from each armpit to join in the middle of his chest and from there followed a straight path to the pubic bone. A steady stream of water washed the blood to a drain at the end of the table. The rib cage had been removed and lay like a discarded jacket next to the body. Two pathology residents were examining the surface of the heart and great vessels.

Looking at the heart lying in the chest, one sees the surface of the right ventricle, the pump that sends venous blood to be reoxygenated by the lungs, and the great vessels that convey the pumped blood to its destination. The left ventricle, which pumps blood out through the aorta, is mostly hidden beneath its companion. The pulmonary trunk emerges from the right ventricle as a short, wide vessel about three centimeters in diameter. It is only five centimeters long and ends in a sharp bifurcation, giving it a T-shape as it sends blood off to each of the nearby lungs. If this trunk were to become occluded, the supply of blood to the brain, the coronary arteries, and the rest of the body would be stopped almost instantaneously. It is possible for large clots of venous blood to form in the deep veins of the leg, break loose, and travel along like chunks of moss in a stream—into the inferior vena cava, the right atrium, through the tricuspid valve into the right ventricle, and out the pulmonary trunk where suddenly they hit a sharp turn and lodge. Pulmonary emboli kill fifty thousand Americans each year.

The resident's knife slit into the base of the glistening white trunk and gently cut out to its bifurcation. She retracted the arterial wall to discover a massive red-black clot, nodular and irregular, like the gnarled root of a bush. Mr. Webster had died of a classic *saddle embolus*. The pathologist tore out four separate emboli that filled virtually the entire lumen of the trunk and both pulmonary arteries. How curious it sounded to hear her words.

"That's a beauty, the best I've seen this year."

I glanced at Mr. Webster's face. It was him alright, but it bore little resemblance to the gentle, dignified man I had talked to yesterday afternoon. The head was turned sharply to the right, the eyes were staring blankly, and a dirty, torn glove draped the left cheek. The tongue hung out, dangling in the bloody water. I was numb; I wanted to feel sad, to mourn for Mr. Webster, but no emotion like that was in me. Death was an awesome fact; like the sun, it overwhelmed. Here in the harsh reality of the morgue I had gotten the knowledge I was after. Now, it was time to go. By the time I had climbed the seven flights of stairs I was almost eager to report my findings to the residents.

The nine-person team that managed the care of the thirty-odd patients on G3W functioned smoothly despite a hectic schedule. The patient population changed every day. Every two weeks one or more members of the team would rotate to a different part of the medical center. Every weekday was chock full of meetings: Right after "work rounds" the residents gave "morning report" to the chief of the service; three mornings a week at eleven-thirty our attending physician, a talented young pulmonary specialist, led a discussion of patient management; and a radiology conference was held each day at three o'clock. It seemed that everyone had so much to do that no one could possibly keep track of all the patients on the service. That is, of course, unless one was a master of "rounds," the time-honored activity with which doctors start their day.

I am tempted to call "morning rounds" a movable feast. Between seven-fifty and eight o'clock we stumbled into the MICU, at least half of us clutching styrofoam cups of tepid coffee and an odd assortment of doughnuts and sweetrolls from the cafeteria two floors below. These would gradually disappear as we moved around the unit and then out onto the general ward. By eight-fifteen most stomachs were quiet, most hands were free, and most attentions were finally focused.

The object of morning rounds is to monitor the management and progress of every patient on the service. The team assembles in a tight circle outside the patient's room. Then the intern who admitted the patient either presents the medical story to the team (if the patient is brand new to the service) or provides a brief update on his care. After the presentation and a few quick questions, the whole team troops in to say hello and assess the patient. If a person is really sick, a brief physical examination and more discussion as to the next course of action usually take place. At the least, the visit forces the doctors to make contact with the patient and give him an opportunity to make comments or ask questions. These sessions rarely last more than a few minutes per patient. But, even at that rapid rate, the residents' unending task is to hurry the team through rounds so they can finish in less than two hours and make it on time to morning report.

The sociology of morning rounds deserves an entire book unto itself. Behavior at rounds is more elaborate than the signal dances of honey bees. As the team moves from room to room one person endlessly replaces another, stepping forward like a soloist in a collegiate singing group "to present." In seconds the team's mood may change from ponderous sobriety to manic hilarity depending on the wit with which a particular intern is endowed. But the mood shifts within the team huddle are not nearly as dramatic as those that mark the interaction between the doctors and the individual patients. For example, I remember one week when four adjacent single rooms housed, in turn, a delightful, intelligent old man dying horribly of pancreatic cancer; a surly heroin addict, who had infected himself by shooting up, and who would not speak to us; a huge, somewhat retarded, laxative abuser, whose room constantly smelled of feces; and a witty con man with COPD, an admitted pickpocket, who was always asking the team to step a little closer to the bed. Needless to say, we apportioned our attentions very differently among these four men. We could do little for the old man, but he got our time and our sympathy. We easily cured the addict with a long course of antibiotics, but we barely looked at him. Hardly anyone ever entered the laxative abuser's room (except to hunt for the laxatives he was constantly stashing), and we regularly bantered with the pickpocket, who always had a joke to tell.

As second-year students we had not been to many "rounds," but we had heard a lot about "roundsmanship." To the outsider, roundsmanship is a mysterious and subtle activity that defies description. As the neophyte participates day after day, however, it becomes much less subtle. Indeed, it acquires the trappings of a challenging game. The skillful player must have the memory of an IBM 360 computer, the erudition of a Talmudic scholar, the poise of a fencer, the wit of a stand-up comic, and an instinct for the jugular.

The basic goal of roundsmanship is to "look good." The students must look good to everyone else, the interns must look good to everyone except the students, and the residents need only look good to the attending physician.

Some attendings, especially the powerful full professors, automatically looked good. On the other hand, young attendings, despite their authority, also had to try to look good to everyone so that they could acquire a reputation that someday would make them automatically look good.

Depending on the level at which you play, there are different ways to look good. The third-year medical student had to satisfy the following minimum requirements: dress neatly, always carry white unlined three-by-five index cards containing all lab results of all patients whom you are following, always look at the house officer who is speaking, ask no less than one but no more than three questions during rounds, never answer a question first unless it is clearly intended for you, never appear to be competing with fellow students, and never challenge a resident's wisdom, especially if you know he or she is wrong and you are right. For extra credit one should always carry unobtrusively some blank index cards, pens, a pocket flashlight, gauze pads, and sterile tongue blades (this list changes when one is doing a surgical clerkship). Adherence to these rules does not guarantee success, but it prevents abject failure. It promises that one will not be branded as an incompetent early in one's career.

For the student who has sufficient intelligence and self-control to master the basics, there are a nearly infinite number of more subtle skills to master. Perhaps the most crucial task is to hone the ability to answer the esoteric questions posed by senior players—not an easy feat. The questions come suddenly and without warning, and there is little hope of knowing the correct answer. Thus style counts a great deal, and it is crucial to pay attention; nothing is worse than to be caught daydreaming. One cannot outgrow this embarrassment. (I once saw a famous gastroenterologist caught napping at a hospital conference. When he confessed that he had been "wool gathering," nervous laughter rained down upon him.) If the question is posed directly to you and you have no idea, do *not* guess. Wait no more than five seconds and say simply, "I'm not sure." This strategy is far superior to the wild guess, for it demonstrates caution and reflection. If the question is tossed to the crowd or to someone else who has missed it, you have an opportunity to look good. This requires an instant assessment of your odds of being right. The best question on which to gamble an answer, assuming you have some basis for a guess, is the "percentage" question. For example, the senior resident asks, "What percentage of patients get gastrointestinal side effects from indomethacin?"—arguably an important fact given the vast quantities of this anti-inflammatory drug prescribed each year. In answering any percentage question, the key numbers that should run through your head are 20, 40, and 80. Just by assessing the nature of the question, you can "fit" one of these best guesses to it. In this case it's easy. A drug that caused discomfort in 80 percent of its users would have little chance on the market. But given the fact that the resident bothered to ask the question, side effects must be common. So is it 20 or 40? Forty is still very high, so try 20. Bingo! You look good. Even if the correct answer is 10, 20 is close enough to score.

Another good trick is to pursue your reading on one subspecialty, even as you struggle to learn the barest minimum in everything else. If you correctly answer a sufficiently difficult question, one with no room for guessing, you can in seconds erase a string of recent errors. I shall never forget the early days of my first medical clerkship, when I squirmed in embarrassment as I missed question after question fired at me by my imperious chief resident. Finally, one day at rounds, with the entire team assembled, he asked us, "What biochemical disease mimics Marfan's syndrome?"

I could barely contain myself. I waited as five seconds of silence ticked by. Then I piped up, "Homocystinuria."

He nodded as all heads turned to me. We were at a cusp. Would he pursue the exchange? He did. "How do you tell them apart?"

This time there was no need for me to wait. "In Marfan's syndrome the lens [of the eye] subluxes up, in homocystinuria it subluxes down." I had him cold. I *looked good!* I could feel my stock rising in the room.

During the medical clerkship the student is "on" with an intern every fourth day. These are the days and nights that he or she gets to "work up" patients. The student is usually the fourth person to do a history and physical exam on the poor patient during the first six hours of hospitalization. (The student exam comes after those performed by the doctor working in the emergency room, the intern, and the admitting resident.) Besides helping the intern by "running scut" (seeking out x-ray reports, gram staining sputum, and other unsavory tasks) most of the night, the student also must read about the patient's illness in order to sound semi-intelligent at rounds the next morning.

One of the milestones in the life of medical students is the first time that they present at rounds. As an anxiety-laden event, this experience ranks somewhere between losing your virginity and skydiving. The first patient that I worked up to present was an unpleasant little man named Clarence Bodmer.

Mr. Bodmer was a fifty-three-year-old crane operator, the father of four children, and a lifelong resident of Waterbury. He had been "well" until nine days earlier, when while walking to the store he had experienced sudden, crushing chest pain and shortness of breath and had fainted. He was taken to a local hospital and admitted in order to rule out a myocardial infarction (a "ROMI" in the trade). All studies were negative, but on his fifth day in the hospital he had experienced another episode of severe chest pain, this time radiating down the left arm. An EKG taken during this episode showed signs of reduced blood flow ("flipped T's in leads V_2–V_6"). After he had another bout of pain the next day, he was transferred to the VA to undergo cardiac catheterization.

Talking with Mr. Bodmer, I gradually began to understand the dimensions of his cardiac disease. He had anginal chest pain since 1970. In 1976 he had undergone a "cabbage," a triple coronary artery bypass graft, because those vessels were so clogged that the heart could not get enough blood to its own muscle. After this heart operation his chest pain had disappeared completely for several years, but now it was back. Mr. Bodmer could not talk enough about his chest pain. It had plagued him for six years and now it was threatening him again. He worried constantly: When would the heart attack come? He spoke like a spoiled child, shifting from angry criticism of his chest surgeons, "who probably botched the first job" to a simpering plea that I help him.

As I examined him, the lessons learned from my second-year practice sessions evaporated. I tried to keep calm and do a systematic head-to-toe exam while we talked, but it was hopeless. Although my memory of this particular physical exam has faded now, I still have the write-up that I handed into my resident for evaluation. The litany of findings I neglected to note is embarrassingly long. In the HEENT exam (head, eyes, ears, nose, throat) I forgot to measure the size of the pupils and their reaction to light, look for nystagmus (a staccato motion of the eyes), check the oral mucosa, examine the neck for nodes or the thyroid for nodules. In the cardiac exam I neglected to note the PMI (point of maximum impulse), describe the second heart sound, mention the absence of murmurs and rubs, note the presence or absence of jugular venous distention (JVD), or comment on the quality of the carotid pulse. My neurological exam was essentially nonexistent. The conclusion was obvious. I could not yet talk to and examine a patient at the same time.

At two o'clock in the morning, after a desperate attempt to write up the patient, learn the drugs used to treat angina, study electrocardiography, memorize the admission laboratory values, and practice presenting Mr. Bodmer's case to a bathroom mirror, I went home to sleep. Six hours later I was standing in the crowded CCU, with my eight team members so close to me I could smell their aftershave lotions, waiting to present. Carol gave me the go ahead. Just as it had in high school when I burst out of the starting blocks to run the 440 yard dash, an immense sense of freedom engulfed me. For the next four minutes I told the world everything I knew about Clarence Bodmer: his pain, his operation, his occupation, his chest scars, his smoking habits, his children, his serum potassium, and his future (a cardiac catheterization tomorrow). Before I knew it I was done. "Excellent job," said Carol. "Let's go see him." Mercifully, no one had challenged me on anything. I had soloed without crashing.

I owe a lifelong debt to the people who were my patients in the VA hospital. During my four years of training I attended hundreds of lectures, read thousands of pages, and walked the hospital corridors with dozens of physicians. No doubt all these experiences were helpful, but my most important teachers were about fifty aging, mostly down and out vets who I saw on G3W. They knew of course that I was a rank beginner, a complete novice, quite definitely not yet a doctor. Every time I entered a patient's room to draw blood, start an IV, or get a blood "gas," he knew from a glance at my white coat (which was ten inches shorter than the intern's coat) that there was a fair chance that I had not yet mastered the procedure and that he was my guinea pig. Even when I was forthright about my amateur status and gave them an opportunity to object, these men rarely complained. Time and again patients said to me, "Do what you have to, Doc; I know you're trying your best."

I remember one old gent with special clarity. Like so many vets, he had smoked heavily for many years. He was now a victim of emphysema; there was barely enough functional lung tissue to suck in the air he needed to live. After coming down with a bad bronchitis he had *decompensated*, and we were treating him with oxygen and antibiotics. We were monitoring his progress with arterial blood gas studies. The test sounds simple enough. A small heparinized needle is poked gently into the radial artery in the wrist below the thumb. The pressure head in the artery drives the blood up the syringe. A special machine analyzes the blood to determine the partial pressure of oxygen and carbon dioxide and its acidity—all indicators of how well the body is being oxygenated.

The radial artery, just a few millimeters below the surface, is usually quite easy to palpate. In fact the first five times I tried to draw a blood gas I was successful. So, when I marched into Mr. Dobzhansky's room, armed both with syringe and experience, I was pretty confident. As I had been taught, I hyperextended his wrist, resting it on a towel, carefully felt the pulse, swabbed the skin with alcohol, and checked the needle's bevel to make sure it was aimed upstream. Quickly, I poked the needle through the skin. He winced but did not move. He knew the worst of the pain was already over. But no bright red blood climbed up the glass walls of the syringe. I gently maneuvered the needle, feeling for the artery. No luck. Would Mr. Dobzhansky let me try again? He nodded. The second effort was no better. I knew that I was doing everything right, but I could not get blood. The sweat was beginning to drip from my forehead, and my hand was starting to shake. Again, I withdrew. This time I apologized to Mr.

Dobzhansky, took off my coat, rolled up my sleeves, and vowed one more try. Again, he assented. Again I felt the artery pumping at my finger. I plunged the needle firmly into this pulse and got back nothing. Defeat. Three sticks in a row had failed. What if this were an emergency? I felt totally incompetent.

I could tell by looking into his eyes that Mr. Dobzhansky's wrist was hurting. Still, he did not complain. I was obviously more upset than he.

"Sit down, son," he said. "Take a break. Get your nerve back. You can do it. It's just a bit tricky."

Suddenly, it was like a boy with his grandfather. All pretense fell away.

"You're right," I said. "Thanks."

So, we talked for awhile about his family. He showed me his son's picture and told me about his heroism in Vietnam. Then, as though he had been timing things, he looked at his watch:

"Let's go. I think you'll get that artery this time."

He calmly talked me through a procedure he had probably undergone fifty times. "Don't plunge that needle in until you're sure. Relax. Take your time."

I did and I was rewarded. Bright red blood slowly filled the syringe.

"Good job," he said. "Thanks a lot."

It was also at the VA that I learned how to perform a lumbar puncture, better known as an LP or spinal tap. Again, this procedure sounds simple enough. The patient is positioned on his side at the edge of the bed. Using a sterile technique, a long needle is guided between the lower spinal bones and the surrounding ligaments and into the canal that houses the nerves. A few cc's of fluid are then drawn off and studied, usually to determine if that space is infected with bacteria. The spinal tap is not a dangerous procedure, but it can be painful (even when the skin is properly anesthetized), and it does carry a small risk of doing great harm (by introducing bacteria that cause meningitis or by dropping the pressure in the spinal column and herniating the brainstem). Medical students regard the LP with some discomfort. It is a tricky procedure. Most people, especially arthritic, obese old men, do not have a nicely curved vertebral column with wide spaces between the spinous processes. One often stabs in the dark.

I shall never forget my first successful "tap"—successful, that is, in terms of obtaining the spinal fluid. Along with Dave Holmes, a bright but angry young intern, I was "following" Robert Steal. The "man of steel," as we called him, was a fifty-year-old alcoholic who looked much more than his real age and was suffering from a profound loss of memory. A CAT scan had shown marked changes inside his brain (predominantly, a loss of tissue), and we thought he had Alzheimer's disease. Nevertheless, an LP was an appropriate part of the workup, and David, a budding neurologist who wondered whether Mr. Steal might have a rare "slow virus" disease, was eager to get some fluid.

Of course the patient was much too out of it to consent to a lumbar puncture. He spent his days sitting hunched up in a chair in silence. Each time I spoke to him I tried to remind him where he was, but minutes later he would not be able to tell me. He frequently thought he was on Grant Street, a place where he had lived decades earlier. He recognized his wife only about half the time, often calling her by his sister's name. After we had explained the purpose and dangers of the LP to her, Mrs. Steal signed the consent form.

Later that night, when more pressing work was finished, David and I grabbed a "spinal kit" and went to Mr. Steal's room. Although it was pointless, we carefully explained the procedure to him, positioned him, and set up the sterile field. With luck an LP takes only a few minutes. The key is to get the patient in just the right position and keep him there. After cleaning the skin and injecting some lidocaine, one inserts a long thin needle between overlapping spinous processes and through the soft tissues. Ideally, one starts on a point midway between the top of the hips and takes imaginary aim at the belly button. When the fluid begins to drip from the collar of the needle it is collected into several tubes, and you are finished.

David had not spent nearly as much time as had I with Mr. Steal. Thus, he was not quite as concerned about his inability to cooperate. Holding Mr. Steal down with one hand, he talked me through the tap. Everything went well and I was collecting the third of four tubes when suddenly, without making a sound, Mr. Steal stood up. As he did the manometer, a thin tube with a stopcock that is routinely used to measure the pressure of the fluid in the spinal canal, crashed to the floor. David had been kneeling next to me, and we were in the fluid's path as it spurted out. I felt it hit my lips and saw it hit David right in the eyes. As David let out a howl, Mr. Steal started to lie down with a four-inch needle in his back. Instinctively, I grabbed and pulled it out, just in the nick of time.

It had all happened in three seconds. Well, I thought, no harm done, and we got the fluid. Wrong! David was dancing up and down in a rage, screaming at his patient.

"You lunatic! Are you trying to kill me?"

For a moment I thought he was going to hit the man. I dragged him into the corridor.

"Take it easy. What's wrong?"

"You don't have to worry, it only hit your lips. But that stuff hit me in the eyes. If he really does have a virus in there, it could be on its way to my brain now," moaned Dave.

The so-called slow virus diseases, such as Creutzfeldt-Jakob disease, are very rare, but very deadly. Slowly, but surely, the viruses destroy the brain. Of course the odds of this happening are very slim, but for the rest of my life I shall wonder if Mr. Steal had a slow virus disorder.

During my six-week stint on G3W I rode the sharpest learning curve of my life. Physicians taught me how to look for clinical signs of illness and which tests to order to decide a differential diagnosis, nurses taught me more basic but critically important tasks such as how to "straight-cath" patients who could not urinate, and patients taught me about suffering and death. One truth I captured at the VA was that every person uniquely handles his own illness. Some people are stoics; other folks whimper. Some people die so quietly that no one notices; others die in agony. We all know these facts to be true, but it is quite incredible to relearn them by being there. A handful of experiences stand out most vividly.

Perhaps the most frightening moment of my medical clerkship came during my first night on call. It had been a quiet evening, the intern had gone to bed and I was about to go home, when the call came from the emergency room that a new patient needed to be admitted to the intensive care unit. I was dispatched on an errand by the intern, and when I returned Mr. Sartini was already in the unit. He was a great whale of a man, weighing at least three hundred pounds, and his arms and legs spilled off the bed, pushed away by his massive belly. He was propped up, nearly sitting, and under the cold glare of the fluorescent light I could see the sweat on his brow and the fear in his soft brown eyes.

He was a "GI bleeder," an alcoholic with a portal hypertension that had caused the veins along his esophagus to dilate massively. A few hours earlier one had ruptured, and he had been vomiting blood ever since. He had been in the ICU before, and he knew these bleeds could kill him. The look of a man wondering if he is about to die is easy to figure out. Despite all of modern medicine there was not much to offer him. The doctor in the emergency room had dropped an "N-G tube." It gave constant access to the source of his bleeding. I tiptoed cautiously behind the nurse, a bluff, no-nonsense woman whom I liked, and watched. On the table next to the bed was a huge basin filled with saline and ice; on the floor were buckets filled with huge clots of blood floating in a foul, brownish liquid. The nurse, armed with a bulb syringe, was intermittently forcing about a cup of iced saline into Mr. Sartini's stomach and then sucking it back up.

About ten seconds after I reached the bedside a technician arrived with two bags of blood, which the nurse was going to run in to Mr. Sartini. "Here, Phil," she said, thrusting the syringe at me. "Would you please take over?" So there I stood with Mr. Sartini, whose constant low-pitched moan was like some horrible muzak, sucking clots of blood from his stomach. For the first thirty seconds I prayed I would not vomit. I remember about then glancing over at John, the senior resident. He sat calmly at the nursing station, as the intern prepared to insert a *CVP line* under his guidance. Here it was nearly two in the morning, there was blood all over the sheets, I was sweating like crazy, and John looked as calm as a bank president reading the *Wall Street Journal*. No doubt my turmoil showed. I remember thinking, as I saw the slightest trace of a bemused smile cross his face, that there was simply no chance: I could never be as in control and confident as he seemed. An hour later Mr. Sartini was stable. Blood and Ringer's lactate were running into his arms, the CVP line was in place, and he had stopped bleeding. Just as the gastroenterologist arrived to "scope him" (put a tube down to identify the bleeding source), I stumbled off to bed, wondering if I had the nerve to be a doctor.

About a week later, during rounds, I saw a man die for

the first time. The MICU is a large open room with eight beds; a pleasant spot on sunny mornings. Shafts of bright white light crisscross the green floor, and from the windows one can sneak a spectacular view of Long Island Sound. I was seduced by the beautiful August morning; as one of the interns discussed a patient whose status had not changed in several days, I glanced about the room. Suddenly, I noticed the monitor hanging over the patient in bed four. The electrical signal that displayed the QRS complex, the signature made each time the heart beats, was markedly slow. Normally, about an inch separated one QRS from another, a pattern consistent with a heart rate of about 70, but at least two inches spaced this man's QRS complexes. I did not know much, but I did know that a heart rate of 35 was trouble.

I was at the outer fringe of a huddle of white coats so I quickly grabbed one of the nurses.

"Look at that monitor over bed four," I said.

"Yes, it looks like he's on his way out now. He's riddled with cancer and he's a DNR. We are not going to do anything." DNR means "do not resuscitate." No one was going to lift a finger while the man in bed four died.

As the team proceeded from one bed to another I could barely follow them. My eyes were locked on that monitor, watching some stranger's heart stopping work. He lay there face up, wrapped to his neck with a white blanket. A shock of white hair covered his forehead. His eyes were closed. There was no sign of struggle. Within ten minutes his heart had slowed to a rate of twenty beats per minute. This was clearly the end. Something seemed terribly wrong to me. A dozen healthy, presumably compassionate young doctors and nurses were within twenty feet of this man. A few had glanced at the monitor, but nobody had said anything. Should not somebody go to this man and offer the warmth of a hand to him in his dying moment? Maybe even in his silence he cried out for comfort. I wanted to go to him, but I was paralyzed. What stopped me? Had the monitor signal so mesmerized me that I was frozen to the final countdown? Was I afraid of acting unprofessionally? Was I afraid to approach death too closely?

I stood pondering the monitor. Only two QRS complexes moved across the screen. Then one. Again one. None. The line went flat. It was 8:38 A.M. The stranger was dead. Nothing changed. He did not look different. No one moved to cover him. I whispered a silent good-bye.

One of the most difficult lessons for medical students to learn is to be totally honest about their impression of a patient. Walking into a world where *everyone* knows more than you do, it is easy to fall into the trap of "finding" a clinical sign, an enlarged liver for example, because you *think* it is supposed to be there. Missing an obvious clue can be quite embarrassing, but embracing ignorance is much better for you and your patients than pretending it does not exist. Another even tougher lesson is that, despite all your ignorance, you must learn to trust yourself. One night in my third week on G3W an old black lady, a World War I nurse, drove those lessons home for me.

She was eighty-two years old and had a multitude of medical problems, including bad emphysema and congestive heart failure. I was not too familiar with her background, but I knew that all her liver function tests were abnormal and that she was under hepatitis precautions. All persons going into Irma's room had to wear gown, gloves, and mask to protect themselves. About ten o'clock, when our other work was finished, Dave and I went down to her room to get a stool sample for culture. Suitably gowned, we went in and found a frail little woman lying uncomfortably in bed. She was running a slight temperature and had a disheveled look. As David was doing a rectal exam, the

nurse who was taking vital signs came to the doorway.
Since we were already gowned, she asked us to take Irma's
blood pressure and pulse. David, utterly convinced (and
with some fairly good evidence) that this particular nurse
was lazy, refused, but I agreed, thinking that her request
made sense. Why soil another gown?

I put the blood pressure cuff around her right arm, my
stethoscope over her brachial artery, pumped the cuff up,
let the air gradually out, and listened. The needle kept
dropping: 100, 90, 80, 70, 60; still, I heard nothing. "What
a dope," thought I, "you can't even take a blood pressure
yet." I tried again. No luck. Feeling quite stupid, I mustered my courage and reported:

"I can't get a BP, David."

Glaring at the nurse, he marched over and took a
pressure himself.

"Eighty over 60. Try again."

I carefully placed my stethoscope in the same spot and
took another reading. Again, no *Korotkoff* sounds. Head
down, I slowly mumbled my lie.

"I agree, 80 over 60."

About an hour later, as I was walking down the corridor,
I heard Irma call out. I quickly donned a gown and went to
her. She was propped up on two pillows and was having a
lot of trouble breathing. She asked me to sit her straight up
and dangle her legs over the side so she could breathe
easier. As I did that, I counted her respiratory rate. She
was breathing fast and working hard at it. With surprising
strength she grasped my arm to control her balance. The
muscles of her neck stood out like whip cords and her
nostrils flared. After gently putting her back in bed, and
reassuring her that I would return, I looked for Dave. He
had been called to see another patient, so I went to the
charge nurse.

"Irma's pretty uncomfortable in her breathing. She
wants to sit up in a chair. Will you help me move her?"

"Oh, that old lady's always complaining. Believe me, she's OK. I saw her ten minutes ago. What she needs is sleep," the nurse replied.

I backed down. Who was I, a green med student, to challenge a nurse twice my age? An hour or so later I finally found David, told him about Irma's breathing difficulty, and said goodnight.

Seven hours later I was back in the hospital. I saw David heading for the cafeteria.

"How was your night?" I asked.

"Terrible. Two patients died. I coded Mr. Einhorn at two A.M., and one of the nurses found Irma dead at four."

A pounding surf of guilt swept over me. My first sin of not arguing that she was hypotensive had been badly compounded when I had not acted more vigorously to alleviate her breathing difficulty. I was angry, too. Had not both David and the nurse been too cavalier about Irma's illness? Perhaps her death could have been prevented. What if an autopsy showed that she died from a cause about which we might have done something? All day long her face floated in and out of my thoughts. Then at about three o'clock I saw David talking to her family. They knew she was quite ill, so death had not surprised them. They refused to sign an autopsy permit, hands were shaken all around, and they left. I would never know what exactly killed her. Later I strolled down to the end of the short corridor where a large window looked down on the quiet little streets of West Haven. As I watched the sun set, I took two vows: Always be honest about what you do or do not find when you examine a patient. If you think a patient is really ill, act on that belief until somebody convinces you that the situation is not dangerous.

In all of medicine, indeed in all of human experience, there may not be any event as dramatic as a "code"—the frantic, all out, no-holds-barred, fourth-and-goal attempt to grab a life from death's clutches. Before I started on the wards, I feared codes much as Henry Fleming, the young recruit in *The Red Badge of Courage,* feared combat. I imagined that there was no challenge that could test me more stringently. There in front of you lies a man whose heart has just stopped beating. Working against horrible odds you have at best a few minutes to start delivering oxygen to his precious brain. Assuming you succeed at that, you have ten or twenty minutes to get the heart beating on its own. There is no room for ignorance, uncertainty, or hesitation. You must act. There is no other way.

There are actually two kinds of codes, and they are vastly different. The typical code, the code you someday become familiar with, begins with a sudden crackle from the loudspeaker. Then comes the strident, repetitive litany: "Code 5, G3W. Code 5, G3W. Code 5, G3W." The harsh metallic call continues, but you don't hear it anymore because you are running hard, and with every step your world is shrinking. Thirty seconds later you are leaping straight into a chaotic universe that is no larger than a hospital room. The more unusual code is the code you call yourself. As you alone work feverishly to revive a dead person, every synapse firing, your heart is tapping out a prayer for help, and the thirty seconds before it is answered are very long.

One night I was sitting in a corner of the dingy dining hall eating dinner with Tim Crowe, my new medical resident, when the loud speaker screamed. Before the message registered in my head, Tim was off and running. I remember racing down the hall and up three flights of stairs, my eyes riveted on his backside, amazed that he could move so fast. As we turned the last corner, nearly colliding with a patient, I saw a nurse opening a "crash cart" by the third door. The code had been called for Mr. Malone. I knew him vaguely. He was a seventy-year-old man with metastatic cancer. In medical parlance he was *cachectic*: The cancer had wasted away his flesh, and he looked like the pictures of prisoners as they marched out of Auschwitz in 1945. But, still, he wanted to live.

There were already three people in the room working on Mr. Malone. Dave was hunched over him with a laryngoscope, a metal blade used to guide a tube through the mouth into the trachea; a respiratory therapist was waiting to "bag breathe" him through the tube that Dave was putting in; and Anthony was kneeling on the edge of the bed pumping Mr. Malone's chest. Automatically, because he was the resident on call that night, Tim started "running the code." He was the general, and his word was law. He started barking orders, and, magically, people kept appearing to carry them out.

With pounding heart, I felt too breathless to do anything. But, the order came: "Phil, get a blood gas. Go for his femoral." I turned toward the crash cart. A wall of people in the hallway formed a tight semicircle around the cart. A nurse thrust a syringe into my hand and held out a thumb-sized bottle of heparin. It was my job to plunge the needle into the rubber top of the bottle and suck back heparin. My hand shook so badly I could not do it. Finally, she grabbed my hand and thrust the bottle into the needle. Quickly, I flushed the syringe and squirted the excess out.

Eight people were now working over Mr. Malone. Someone was starting an intravenous line on one arm. An intern was injecting an "amp of bicarb" into a big leg vein. One nurse was putting EKG leads on his arms and feet; another nurse hovered in a corner with a clipboard, furiously recording everything being done. I dropped to my knees at the edge of the bed. Mr. Malone lay naked, already half covered by paper and used gauze pads. He was so thin that I should have been able to see his femoral artery bulging out of his groin, but this man's heart no longer beat. He had no measurable blood pressure. Still I could feel a certain fullness three finger breadths back from his pubic bone. I plunged the needle straight down. Slowly, blood started inching up the syringe. I drew back to hurry it and quickly handed the sample to the nurse who would run it to the lab. About four minutes had elapsed since the code began, but I had no idea how many had elapsed since he stopped breathing. Four? Six? Ten? Were his brain cells still working? Two minutes could make all the difference.

Tim stood at the EKG monitor. A long, thin, green ribbon of paper dropped down its side and curled slowly along the floor. There was no electrical signal. Whenever the person doing CPR paused, the line was flat. Mr. Malone's heart was simply not helping at all.

"OK," yelled Tim, "let's zap him."

The defibrillator cart had appeared out of nowhere. Someone I didn't know was leaning over Mr. Malone's chest, a paddle in each hand, while a nurse squirted a circle of paste on his right chest and left side.

"OK, everybody off the bed. Hit him!"

In a millisecond the room was silent. The paddles hit the skin. A tiny buzz sounded, and he seemed to lift off the bed like a high jumper trying for the extra inch over the crossbar. His entire body stiffened, reminding me of old gangster movies that showed executions in the electric chair.

Somebody yelled, "We got a rhythm." A ragged line wandered across the EKG monitor paper. It was the signal of ventricular fibrillation. His ventricles were quivering on their own. But it was no victory. "V-fib" is a terminal rhythm. In thirty seconds Mr. Malone's heart lapsed back into electrical silence.

The code lasted forty minutes—a long time especially considering that he was probably dead before it had started. I drew a blood gas every five minutes for twenty minutes. As each set of blood gas values were called in we watched the crucial pH drop lower. It had started at 7.15, indicating severe acidosis. The fourth blood gas was reported at 6.80, compatible only with death. As the code progressed, one could detect the shift in attitude. Although everyone still worked, the possibility of survival was extremely remote. The interns dropped out of the game, and the medical students were suddenly more involved. I was sent to the CCU to get a "transthoracic pacer," a special electrode on a long needle that can be jammed into the heart to try to start it up again. Sprawled over Mr. Malone as though they were wrestling, Tim placed the pacing needle correctly on his first try, and people murmured their congratulations. But the heart still did not beat. Even to my unpracticed eye this seemed to be a futile gesture. About five minutes after the pacer wire went in, Tim ended the code.

"That's it, folks. Thanks for coming. You did well."

The hallway crowd had already dispersed. About eight people wandered out of the room down the corridor, breaking quickly into twos to review the last half-hour of their lives. It is the kind of experience that a beginner just cannot walk away from. You relive it four or five times that night and maybe once or twice that week before you file it away. Of course, if it is your first code, if there have not yet been so many deaths that they crowd each other out of your brain, you put it on a special shelf of the memory box along with those other unforgettable moments.

In seconds the room was quiet. I stood alone by the thin, ashen body, letting the scene burn into my memory. Mr. Malone lay naked, his pale blue eyes staring at the ceiling. A tiny rivulet of dried blood ran from one corner of his open, toothless mouth down his neck. He wore a look of angry disbelief. His dentures lay in a crevice between his neck and the pillow. The transthoracic wire jutted out of his chest. The bed and the floor were littered with detritus of a code: gauze pads, needle containers, empty plastic ampules of cardiogenic drugs. The blood-stained sheet was crumpled in a corner. A small plastic container of orange juice had spilled from the bedside table onto his belly. The hallway light gave it a sticky, glistening look. The EKG electrodes, tiny bits of metal fastened to rubber straps, still ran from the machine to his wrists and ankles. The room looked like a writer's image of a modern torture chamber.

It had not occurred to me to ask what happens to a patient after he dies. Who takes him to the morgue? Surely, it was a nursing job, but no nurse was about. It seemed unfair for all of us to have left Mr. Malone just lying there in the mess we had made. It would take just a few minutes to clean the place up. I gently pulled out the chest wire and then removed the electronic shackles from his wrists and ankles. I brushed the various tubes and needles and pads from the bed to the floor. A small white towel lay in the sink. I wet it and quickly wiped the blood off his face and juice off his belly. I shook out the sheet and covered him to the neck. Then I turned his head away from the harsh hallway light so that his dead eyes could look out the window at the stars.

Although I learned a lot of medicine and a great deal about death during my six weeks at the VA hospital, the most important lessons I learned were about what it means to be a patient. During the first year of medical school we had taken a highbrow course called The Behavioral Basis for Medical Care. In it we had read the work of Talcott Parsons, who argued that a powerful set of psychological and cultural forces shape the interactions between doctor and patient. He asserted that the "sick role" carried with it a set of rights and responsibilities distinctly different from those we observe when we are well. As I walked the wards and talked with patients, I realized how profoundly one's life changes upon entering a hospital.

Mr. Harbranch taught me about the bitter frustration

one feels as one loses control of life. He was an eighty-five-year-old World War I veteran who had been a moderately successful meat wholesaler. A couple of minor strokes had crippled him, and he was now living with his niece. He had fairly severe emphysema so that any bout of pneumonia earned him a trip to the VA hospital. I met Mr. Harbranch shortly after he had been admitted to the MICU. Being the medical student on call, I had the right (or duty, I was never sure which) to work him up. Because I was usually the fourth examiner, I was used to patients' resisting my efforts, but nothing had prepared me for Mr. Harbranch.

"Hello, Mr. Harbranch, my name is Philip Reilly, and I am one of the people who will be taking care of you."

He glared back for a moment, then he spoke. "Get the hell out of here."

"I can't do that, Mr. Harbranch. It is my job to get to know you and examine you."

"God damn it. I have been poked all afternoon. I'm sick of it. Leave me alone. Get out!"

I had been instructed to be firm. I drew the curtain around the bed, opened my little black bag, and tried to look like I meant business.

"Mr. Harbranch, I know you've been poked about. I will be as brief as possible. This is for your own good."

This was a lie. The exam was solely for my benefit.

He said nothing, but rolled a few inches away from me. Thinking his silence conveyed a small measure of compromise, I put my stethoscope to his chest and told him I was going to listen to his heart. I had just closed my eyes to concentrate better on the heart sounds when I took a stinging blow to the right cheek. My glasses went flying into the curtain and fell to the floor. Mr. Harbranch hated me with his eyes.

"Now, damn it, get out!"

He had mustered his last ounce of energy to struggle for a tiny measure of privacy. For one second I felt a tremendous urge to force his arms down and continue my exam. But, what claim did I have on his body? He was a cantankerous goat, but he had his rights.

"As you wish, Mr. Harbranch. I will come by in the morning to visit."

By the next morning Mr. Harbranch's breathing was already improved so he moved to a bed on the floor. At rounds I took a few jibes about my bedside manner, but everyone agreed that this was a straightforward case and that our unfriendly patient would soon go home. I visited him that afternoon, hoping that by bringing him the good news that his stay would be short, we might get on a bit better. I did not have much luck at first, so I went to my secret weapon. I had learned early that vets, especially World War I vets, loved to tell war stories. Even with Mr. Harbranch, it worked. After a bit of persuasion he proudly told me that he had won a Purple Heart for wounds suffered while leading an infantry attack on a German machine gun. Later he had been hit with mustard gas and suffered severe lung damage. After talking for about fifteen minutes I asked if I could listen to his breathing.

"Yes, but first get me my clothes. There is no reason why I have to lie around in this damn johnny-coat all day."

"But, Mr. Harbranch, why do you want to wear clothes in bed?"

"That is none of your business, sonny."

Sensing that I was soon to lose the few yards that I had gained, I told him that I would ask the nurse to get his clothes as soon as I examined him. I felt like a parent trying to convince a child to eat dinner. I knew the nurses would not dress him. That was against the unspoken rules that defined the sick role. Patients do not wear street clothes; they have their own uniforms.

It was on the third day after Mr. Harbranch's admission that Roy Kaback, the intern in charge of caring for him, told me that the niece, a strident woman in her fifties, had just telephoned to say that she was going to Florida for two weeks and that he would have to stay in the hospital until her return. She had dumped him on us, and there was nothing we could do about it. Despite the clarity with which he objected to my behavior, Mr. Harbranch had long periods of disorientation, especially at night (a phenomenon in elderly patients called "sundowning"). It was very difficult to explain to him why he had to stay in the hospital for two more weeks.

As each day passed, things became more difficult. I would visit him at about four o'clock to try to talk with him and examine him. By the end of the first week the ritual was well established. After I greeted him, he would glare at me for a few minutes without speaking. Then, as I would try to readjust the nasal prongs that brought him oxygen, he would slap at my hand and roll away. I would ask: "Is there anything I can do for you, sir?" "Leave me alone, I just want to die."

Mr. Harbranch told me this nine times in the next nine days. When I left the service for my next rotation, he was still on the floor, and we were still waiting for his niece to return from Florida.

A certain protocol governs the interactions between patients and doctors in the typical community hospital. The patients are middle class and usually well insured. The doctors are well-heeled and carry a manageable patient load. Both groups are well mannered and, except under the most egregious circumstances, they interact politely, if not cordially. At the VA hospital, this atmosphere of diplomacy was much thinner. The patients were mostly from the lower economic strata, many were pensioners of the government, and a significant percentage were alcoholics. For the most part they were cared for by residents and students. Not a few suspected (erroneously) their treatment was second class, and this belief shaped their conduct toward the house staff.

At first glance the dynamics at the VA hospital did not seem unusual to me, but I gradually saw that these patients were very streetwise and quite manipulative. They were genuinely grateful for good care, but they were quick to note their objections to things they did not like. They knew that they could rarely beat the system, but they still derived pleasure from poking fun at it. I soon realized that the patients, all former enlisted men, perceived us as green, young officers and that they obeyed their orders with a mocking gleam in their eye.

Their attitude became really apparent when I started eavesdropping during rounds. Each morning we trooped in to visit the men in their four-bedded barracks. Despite the early hour, they were usually all up and waiting for us—a gaggle of ten doctors and students. As we moved from one bed to the next, I noticed that the three patients who were not being confronted were watching us like hawks. We were not an impressive sight. At any given moment at least two team members were glancing out the window, watching the news on the overhead televisions or chatting. On some occasions a few team members would be leaving a bedside before the rest even got there. One day I heard a patient joke that we looked like a busload of tourists bored with the exhibits in that room.

While I was on G3W, we discovered the existence of the "bathroom club." At about ten o'clock each morning a clique of patients would begin to fill the large men's room at one end of the corridor. Its attractions were obvious: The windows caught the morning sun, smoking was permitted, and the staff would not overhear them. The extra wheelchairs were stored here, so frequently they would set them up and pass the morning in a metallic circle discussing their ailments, their doctors, and the system. The club members were constantly changing, but since many vets were in no rush to leave the hospital and because some were masters of the extended stay, I was able to identify the regulars. The club's hero was a forty-five-year-old taciturn, surly heroin addict named Melvin. He had a heart murmur so loud that you could hear it without a stethoscope. It was widely rumored that he shot up in the bathroom, but no one ever caught him. He was the hero because he was refusing the surgery his doctors recommended, despite their threat that to do so was a death sentence. The club's mascot was a gigantic, mildly retarded man named John, the confirmed laxative abuser, who had had chronic diarrhea for more than a year. Standing six foot seven and constantly stinking of feces, he was more than any doctor wished to deal with. The only time he changed his pajamas was to attend the club meetings, where he would guffaw wildly at any joke made about the hospital.

The club's leader was a red-faced alcoholic named Bill who had logged nearly a month with his problem of unexplained leg pain. At least once a day he had paroxysms of pain that drove him to beg for narcotics. Each time we would decide to discharge him he would miraculously start running an impressive fever. Bill was one of the most manipulative persons I have ever met. He was obsequious to the physicians. His episodes of pain were truly impressive to observe, and his fevers were high. But no one ever found anything wrong with him. He had been admitted to the VA hospital on nine other occasions (always in the winter), and he was extremely knowledgeable about the system. I suspect that he spent a lot of club time coaching other patients on how to provide realistic symptoms to doctors.

It was at the VA that I first learned to pull tricks on patients during the physical examination. I noticed that one of my patients, an old Italian gentleman who was eager to cooperate, had extremely brisk deep tendon reflexes. When I tapped his knee, the foot sprang out. A few minutes later I gently tapped his shin bone and the foot again jumped forward.

"Mr. d'Angelo, I know you are trying to help, but there is no way that my tap on that part of your leg could make it jump, unless you were doing it yourself."

He grinned sheepishly and apologized. Ever since then I put one trick in my exam, just in case.

August flowed into September, and as the maple leaves reddened and fell, "first medicine" ended. On my last day as a med student in G3W, I felt as much sadness as I did relief. For more than two years I had anticipated this moment. However infinitesimal, a part of my clinical training was now receding into the past. It did not seem possible. First medicine demonstrated that one could learn to be a physician. It restored in me a measure of confidence. As I looked forward to other clerkships, I now knew I would take them in stride.

Chapter 6

THE THERAPEUTIC COMMUNITY

The clinical clerkship year is an infinite series of beginnings. Knowing that their year is divided into seven blocks of six-to-nine weeks, each one spent on a different medical planet, third-year students accept that they will never become familiar with these environments. But, as they spin through the rotations, students soon realize that within each time block are an infinite series of new starts. Interns change, attendings come and go, residents rotate, and, most importantly, patients materialize and vanish—all on their own mysterious schedules. The year is a blur of names and faces.

Furthermore, nearly every day third-year students do something—often something quite stressful—for the first time. One busy Saturday night as I was shadowing a surgical resident who had too much to do, he interrupted his suturing of a forehead laceration on a drunken old man and told me to don gloves and finish the job. When I protested that I had never sutured before, he pointed out that was why he had told me to glove. He also reminded me that this particular gentleman's head had been sutured many times and that he was well anesthetized. To my surprise, I sutured him.

I could recount similarly stressful experiences about

learning vein puncture, drawing arterial blood gases, performing lumbar punctures, paracenteses (putting a needle into the abdomen to draw off fluid), electrocardiograms, femoral sticks (drawing blood from the groin), placing urinary catheters, starting intravenous lines, and placing chest tubes (for drainage). I vividly remember that the first time (under close supervision) I used electric paddles to cardiovert (shock) a patient out of an irregular heart rhythm into a normal rhythm, I wondered if I would also need to be cardioverted. All the changes and all the challenges left little time for reflection.

The one quiet harbor in the high seas of the third year was the psychiatry clerkship, a rotation I did in September and October. Although only a few stairs separate the peripatetic world of medicine from the ward on which I was introduced to psychiatry, they were worlds apart. On medicine the background noise had been the steady beep of cardiac monitors; the first sound I hear on the psychiatry ward was an inane disco tune blasting from the stereo in the solarium. On the medical floor, each day began at 7:30 A.M. when we met for rounds. We rushed around the hospital for two hours checking data on old patients and listening to the interns present the new "players" who had been admitted during the night. On the psychiatry service, the staff often did not hear the official presentation of a new patient until several days after admission.

I had been assigned to work with a resident named Jerry Phelps, and I liked him right away. About twenty-eight years old, he had curly brown hair, horn-rimmed glasses, and an impish twinkle in his eye. Looking for all the world like a model in an L. L. Bean catalog, he was a master of the art of casual dressing. He looked better in a plaid shirt, pressed chinos, and moccasins than I could in a three-piece suit. I found him at his desk in the residents' room, clutching a cup of coffee and doodling as he pondered a patient's chart. After I introduced myself, he dropped the chart, showed me where to find the coffee, and, obviously enjoying what he frankly admitted was his first opportunity to play mentor to a medical student, proceeded to orient me.

The "ninety-day unit," I learned, was famous in psychiatric circles as one of the oldest, most thoroughly studied, and successful "therapeutic communities." This term describes a way of operating a psychiatric ward that encompasses and transcends standard treatments such as drug therapy. It is premised on the notion that there should be close relationships between the staff and the patients. It envisions people working together to run a small society and to solve the problems of its citizens. The unit's "constitution" describes the ward as "a community whose goal is that each can learn how to be responsible for himself and is able to help himself through helping others."

To accomplish that therapeutic goal, the patients were plunged into a rigorous schedule of activities that filled their day much as a job or school work occupied their time before their illness. To a newcomer (staff or patient) there were a bewildering array of meetings. Some, such as "small-group therapy," were chaired by one or two staff members whose job it was to guide discussions by several patients about their problems. The "big leaderless" meeting, attended *only* by patients, focused on the "state of the community," a term with which I would grow quite familiar. "Family meetings" were held twice a week, on Wednesday night and Saturday morning. A patient was *not* accepted into the community (admitted to the service) unless his family agreed to attend these sessions, which forced them to share the impact of illness in one person upon his relatives. The communitywide "patient-staff" meeting also took place twice weekly. These were the most tension-filled sessions. Each revolved around a formal agenda composed by those patients who sat on the advisory board. The main topics were "status changes," "passes," and the ominous "items for discussion." During patient-staff meetings one glimpsed the curious pecking order and power struggles between the various patients. This was far more subtle and important than their formally acknowledged place in the community hierarchy, which was largely a function of seniority.

Upon entering the community each patient was placed at the bottom rung of a ladder of privileges known collectively as "status." As time passed and as the new patient completed certain formal tasks such as memorizing community rules and demonstrated to the satisfaction of the other patients and the staff an attempt to help himself or herself *and* others, the patient would be granted incremental increases in privileges. The patient began on "staff special," literally under constant watch by staff members. Usually, unless considered suicidal or floridly psychotic, the patient would quickly be promoted one rung to "patient special." This meant that most of the waking hours would be spent with a more senior patient who could teach him or her the ways of the ward. After proving the ability to "work" in the community, the patient was a candidate for "independent" status. This step meant being able to move alone about the ward within the limits imposed by the general community ordinances.

The next big step was to "buddy." Two buddies were allowed to leave the ward, each shouldering responsibility for the other, for short periods of time. In good weather "buddy walks" were quite popular. Among the patients it was definitely a status symbol to be named a "monitor." The daily monitor was charged with making sure all the patients complied with the various community rules (being on time for breakfast or for their medications). When there were several new patients, this job was demanding. Finally, one could become a member of the advisory board, the small group that gravely considered the status changes and passes requested by the patients, and presented their recommendations to the patient-staff meeting. The long climb from "staff special" to membership on the advisory board took at least thirty days; some of the more troubled patients never reached the top spot.

To succeed in the community patients had to demonstrate they were trying to explore and solve their problems. Because every community member had some say in promotions, patients were constantly being reviewed. As a patient did progress within the community, the system operated naturally to turn personal concerns outward. Once reaching the rank of "independent," a patient was eligible for "passes," short furloughs into the outside world. Patients might then test their ability to interact with family, set up job interviews, or look for an apartment in preparation for eventual discharge.

Of course, patients fared very differently in the therapeutic community. No question, it was a demanding place to "work." Age, intelligence, and chronicity of illness were key factors in limiting the prognosis. There were also the harsh realities of insurance coverage. As covered days (usually about eighty) dwindled, the staff had to arrange the disposition of the patient, regardless of progress. This disposition sometimes came rather suddenly and, especially if involving a "leader," could disrupt the community.

Even in the best of circumstances there were many therapeutic failures. In studying the history of the ward, I learned that researchers had identified three classes of persons—preconverts, converts, and rejectors—for each of which one could calculate different prognostic expectations. These persons were placed into one of these groups by staff consensus on the basis of their "social openness" during their first week on the ward. (This categorization was, of course, not shared with the patient; nor was it intended to be an ironclad ruling.) The preconvert, with high social openness, tended to be less ill and better educated than others. Alice, a college student whose childhood had been complicated by chronic renal disease and many housebound years, had become severely depressed when she learned that she had to undergo a kidney transplant. Her successful upper-middle-class parents had imbued her with the desire to do well, so she was a natural for the system. Within days after joining the ward, Alice became a leader. The convert's behavior also tended to "improve" rapidly, but there was often a delay of a week or two. Converts tended to be more severely ill and less familiar with the upwardly mobile demands of the community. Typically, their family life was fragmented and their sense of trust slow to develop. If staff or patients made the therapeutic connection with them, there was a chance of major progress. The rejectors tended to be older, sicker persons who were socially very isolated. They came to the ward from a world that offered little hope, and few promises awaited them on discharge. Although they usually made some progress, they often slipped rapidly after leaving the hospital. Of course the staff was acutely aware of the limited value of such generalizations, but they had some validity.

The first of the many meetings in which I would participate during my clerkship was the staff meeting held after lunch each Monday. The nurses, social workers, and two residents gathered around a ping-pong table that had been dragged to one corner of the solarium to create an instant conference room. About a minute later the floor chief, Dr. John Banta, mustached, ruddy-faced and horn-rimmed, strode to the only unoccupied chair and dropped a sheaf of papers to the table as though it were a gavel. The meeting had begun. Jerry urged me to observe closely, and I was rewarded. Although I knew nothing about the patients whose "care plans" were being discussed, it took me less than an hour to realize that like the patients the staff was enmeshed in a very subtle web of power relationships. I guessed correctly that slight disagreements over a patient's care sometimes masked major differences in therapeutic philosophy. A little later I realized that these disputes also reflected major disagreements between staff members about the clinical competence of their colleagues.

I do not mean to imply that the staff was seething with discontent. In fact the nurses, family therapists, and physicians were extremely talented people. But they worked in a structure that fostered power struggles. The two residents, both men in their mid-twenties and in their first year of psychiatric training, were the primary therapists for the patients. They would be working on this floor for six months. A chief resident, two years ahead of them in training, offered some guidance. There were also eight psychiatric nurses, several of whom had been working in the therapeutic community for over a decade. Each patient worked with a primary nurse therapist as well as with a physician therapist. Unlike the physicians, the nurses usually had primary responsibility for a single patient. Given that they had many more years of experience and were deeply invested in the floor on which they worked, it was hardly surprising that the nurses might feel that they knew better than the green residents what therapeutic course to steer for particular patients. Similarly, the three family therapists, all trained social workers with decades of experience, could argue that they knew best what troubled the patient. In fact, they often did know the most about the dynamics of a particular family. As the weeks slipped by I would watch my resident struggle with a tough problem. How could he accede to good advice given by a well-intentioned but slightly patronizing nurse or social worker without letting his tenuous hold on the reins of authority slip? This problem surfaced most acutely with a patient of Jerry's named Bob. Mary, the counselor working with Bob's family, used a counseling strategy that contrasted sharply with Jerry's. Somehow I got caught between them.

Bob, a tall, blond, gentle-faced seventeen-year-old, was the most engaging patient on the floor. In a place populated by withdrawn, deeply depressed patients, wild manics, and lots of folks with "borderline personality disorders," he behaved impeccably and radiated intelligence. A few hours after I arrived on the floor he had welcomed me and drawn me into a conversation about the life of a medical student. I remember finding it difficult to believe that he was a patient.

Bob was the second of four teenaged children born to a hard-driving salesman and his wife. On the surface the family was not unlike a million other American families. During the last twenty years the father had climbed the corporate ladder, leaping from one job to another in search of more money and a better home for his kids. About two years earlier he had finally landed a great job and moved the family from Ohio into a large colonial house in a Connecticut suburb. Everything went well for the family in their new home for about a year until Bob's world, the world of an honors student and basketball player, began to crumble. Gradually, the spats between Bob and his brothers and sister took on new dimensions. Minor annoyances began to anger him greatly. An avid reader, Bob became completely intolerant of his brother's stereo. As far as he was concerned, the volume could not be reduced to an acceptable level. He pounded the walls between their bedrooms until Michael turned off the stereo. Dinner table banter, with several conversations going at once, irritated him so much that Bob took to eating in his room. As the football season ended and basketball practice started, he became more withdrawn, quitting the team after a few days. Any disturbance at home was intolerable; at the slightest provocation Bob would stalk out on walks that lasted thirty miles. In November, despite the pleas and threats of his parents, he built a makeshift bedroom in a corner of the basement and became a virtual recluse. A few weeks later, after a violent outburst at school, he joined us.

I first heard Bob describe his feelings at a small group therapy session that Jerry led twice a week. These meetings, run much like AA (Alcoholics Anonymous) meetings, demanded painful honesty.

"My house wasn't what you think," Bob said bitterly. "It was not a nice quiet house in the country. For me it was like Macy's ten days before Christmas. It was crowded everywhere. Everyone was always noisy and always pushing and fighting over nothing. No peace and quiet. Nowhere to go. It was hell. I couldn't stand it. I couldn't breathe. I had to get out."

Bob was hypercritical of his family. He thought that his father was hard and distant, offering the family not love but money. His older brother was a "pothead" with no direction in life, and his younger sister was a "baby," always crying for her own way. His younger brother was a "clown," and his mother let the other kids walk all over her. Bob, who loved great literature, art, and classical music, dreamed of becoming a teacher or a priest. He saw the other children as leading wasted lives. Unfair though it was, I remember that Bob's world view evoked in me images of Hitler's youth corps that I had seen portrayed in some avant-garde movie. He spoke like a dreamy idealist who was quick to anger and act when things did not go exactly as he wished.

As I talked to him outside of regular meetings, I began to see that Bob wanted all human intercourse to operate at the highest level. At times I felt that he totally controlled our "friendship." Typically, he would invite me to his room to discuss some esoteric questions about Kafka's novels or El Greco's paintings. After about twenty minutes he would, like a busy executive (his father?), glance at his

watch and usher me back to the hall. He went about his
days with great purpose. His work as a floor "monitor" was
flawless, and, as he was charged to do, he spent most of his
time talking to patients about their troubles. I never saw
him relaxing in the game room or kidding with his room-
mates.

Until my first "family meeting," I thought Bob was "high
strung" but not terribly ill. Family meetings were held
after dinner on Wednesday. We filled one of the large
bedrooms with about thirty folding chairs arranged in a
circle and waited for the parents (most of our patients were
teenagers) to arrive. Before the meeting the families huddled in little clusters talking in low tones to their kids.
Sharply at eight o'clock Meriam, the nurse who led the
meeting with Jerry, made a few brief announcements.
When she stopped, silence fell like a curtain. Thirty people
stared nervously into space. I could feel my heart beating,
so I used it as a watch and ticked off the seconds, wondering who would break the squirmy silence. A full minute
passed before Bob's father, a big, well-dressed man with
the demeanor of a small-time politician, broke the ice,
launching into a monologue about how he had struggled
with his son's illness during the week. But as he talked, I
began to notice a subtle condescension in his tone. He was
playing up to the staff. I could read his mind: "The doctor
wants us to talk. These dummies can't talk, so I'll get the
ball rolling."

As the hour slipped away, with Jerry, Meriam, and I
hardly speaking (a staff policy), no one tried to wrest
control from Bob's dad. After describing his own feelings,
he began to ask other parents how they dealt with their
guilt and sorrow. In less than twenty minutes he was as
firmly in charge as any psychiatrist, virtually forcing the
other parents to talk. Some wilted under his gaze; others
flowered. About eight-thirty I noticed that Bob was growing very restless, crossing and uncrossing his legs, and

rocking back on his chair. By eight forty-five he was extremely agitated. I could feel him counting the minutes until he could escape. He just made it, bolting out of the room as soon as Meriam halted the meeting at nine o'clock.

Bob's parents had noticed his restlessness, and they hurried to him. I lingered in the corridor outside his room, easily hearing the raised voices. Bob was embarrassed by his father's behavior. Suddenly, he was screaming.

"Can't you stop acting like a jerk?"

From the doorway I saw him punch the wall very hard. There was an audible crunch, and blood flowed. Jerry and Meriam rushed into the room, ushered the parents out, and quickly took a sobbing Bob to the first-aid station. What had gone wrong? I was bewildered.

During the next hour, as we met with Bob and his parents, some of his problems became a little clearer. He hated his father's need to take over every situation. Bob was enraged because he felt that his father would not accept his illness or his need to be under psychiatric care. He had started screaming and punching the wall to "prove" his illness. That punch had abraded Bob's knuckles, but it had hurt his father a lot more. Was that what he had wanted? The meeting ended with a "victory" for Bob; his parents finally agreed to try family therapy with Mary.

During the therapy sessions with Bob's family on the next two Mondays, I got an intense feeling for the pain bubbling just beneath the surface. These sessions also raised grave doubts in me about the dangers of digging too deeply into "family pathology."

Mr. and Mrs. Brierly brought their three other children to the first session. They joined Mary, Jerry, Bob, and me in a cluttered but comfortable little office.

It was Mary's show, and she wasted no time. Bob had complained to her a lot that his brothers antagonized him, so she began the session by challenging them on that score. Michael, the older brother, deftly deflected her attack,

saying that she was exaggerating the situation. So she
shifted her attention to Joey, a gangly fifteen-year-old who
crouched in a corner, looking out the window, obviously
wishing he were somewhere else. When he did not respond, she persisted, blaming him for Bob's problems. For
the moment she was acting as Bob's advocate, and I
watched a vengeful smile steal across his face. But, Mary
seemed to go too far. Unable to deal with her rain of
questions, Joey started sobbing. My first thought was how
fragile he seemed. Then I realized what a strange, difficult
scene this was for a young kid. Some woman he had never
seen before was blaming him for his brother's illness.
Despite Mary's decision to let up on him, he continued to
sob uncontrollably. A moment later his sister was crying
too. Mr. Brierly could no longer stand it. Angrily accusing
Bob of plotting to harm his brother, he ended the meeting
and ordered the children out of the room. Mary and I
waited until the family was on the elevator and Jerry had
taken Bob back to his room. As we walked to the stairs she
told me how pleased she was with the insights she had
gained. I could not believe my ears. I had found her
counseling technique to be hostile and harmful. So, I was
sure, had Bob's family. I was very surprised when they
agreed to return for a second go-round.

The next Monday was a big day for Bob. Like Mary, he
felt that a lot of "progress" had been made during the first
tension-filled meeting. I was not surprised at this. I knew
that Bob did not really believe that talking with other
patients about their problems could help him. He saw
family therapy sessions as his ticket out of the hospital, the
value of which he questioned. Bob thought that it was his
family, not he, who really needed help. As we walked to
the counseling office for the second meeting he was all
smiles, but the second we entered the room I knew that
there would be trouble.

The Brierly family had had a week to ruminate over the

last therapy session. One look at their faces, frozen in hard-edged smiles, told me that they were united by anger and ready for battle. Mary decided to square off with Mr. Brierly at once.

"Ted, I noticed that you and Margaret both missed family meeting last Wednesday. What happened?"

A bomb seemed to explode inside Ted's head. His knuckles went white and his face reddened. His voice shook. "If you think we missed the meeting because we were upset about last Monday, Mary, you're wrong. I missed a plane and Margie was tied up with the kids. But let me tell you something else. We are upset. All of us. We're mad, damned mad at you. What business do you have attacking a fifteen-year-old kid. What counseling school taught you to do that? We don't think you can help us or Bob. And I'll tell you one thing, you are not going to behave again as you did last week."

The power of Ted's outburst had caught Mary off guard. She tried to play it cool and to explain that family therapy sometimes required tearful scenes. But her voice betrayed her. Surrounded by five angry faces, she was obviously nervous. She tried to be conciliatory, but the family was out for revenge. I hung back, trying to disappear into the woodwork. The plain fact was that I sided with Bob's family. I would not want patients of mine to work with Mary. I prayed that she would not call on me as an ally. Of course, she did.

"Phil, do you think I was unfair to Joey last week?"

I tried to calm the waters and yet be honest. "I think Joey was in a tough spot. We could have eased into things more slowly."

"Do you think I was attacking the family?"

I paused. I knew the answer she wanted, but it was not what I believed. What should I do? Though only a fledgling medical student, I had thought a lot about the doctor-patient relationship. Surely, a counseling session should operate on presumptions of honesty and openness between clinicians and families. But would an honest answer cause more harm than a dishonest one?

I had not asked to be put in this dilemma. Having no clinical certainty about how to act, I chose to speak frankly. "Mary, you gave everybody a pretty rough time."

Mr. Brierly lit up in a triumphant glow. He quickly mounted a new verbal attack against Mary. I could sense her anger at me. I had refused to help her stop the attack. Fortunately, a few minutes later the scene dissolved when Jerry, who had been busy with a long-distance call, knocked and entered. The rest of the hour was devoted to peace making. Gradually and against her will, Mary yielded control of the family therapy session to Jerry.

After the session ended I realized that Mary had chosen to blame me for her inability to handle the Brierlys' anger. As we walked to the elevator in embarrassed silence, her eyes tossed daggers at me. At the door she had only one sentence for me.

"That's the last therapy session of mine that you are going to attend."

Before I could reply, she turned and headed for the stairs. Until that evening Mary had been courting me. We had lunched together several times, and she had offered to help train me. In the remaining three weeks of my clerkship she never spoke to me again.

When I left the community Bob's condition had not changed much. He was now certain that the hospital was not going to help him and was pretty eager to leave. But his fears about his ability to live at home remained very strong. The staff was chagrined. The chief psychiatrist had concluded that he was suffering from schizophrenia (of which restlessness and anxiety are cardinal features). Our drugs and milieu therapy hadn't helped him, and everyone feared that his illness would be chronic. There was a very real chance that he would be in and out of psychiatric hospitals for the rest of his life.

My main task on the ward was to work up and present all newly admitted patients to the staff at rounds. In psychiatry the history-taking process is vastly different from that in internal medicine. Compiling as complete a patient biography as possible is a critical task to which one might have to devote many hours of interviewing. One also has to interview family members and read every available record to check the patient's tale. In the process the psychiatrist may uncover some incredible stories, one fascinating aspect of this field. On not a few occasions as I did my workups I felt more like Perry Mason than Sigmund Freud.

Another task that I had to perform was to become familiar with the mental status exam and other more specific questioning techniques. Psychiatrists developed the mental status exam to help them identify the kind of disorder from which a patient suffers. Although the exam involves a distinct set of questions, it really begins the second that a physician walks into the patient's room. With a glance the physician can gather much information about a person's overall state. How is the patient dressed? What is the initial facial expression offered to the interviewer? Fear? Anger? A patient sitting in the corner with her head down triggers a vastly different set of concerns than does a patient who strides forward to shake hands with the interviewer. The quality of speech is also exceedingly important. Does the patient talk freely and easily? Are there any unusual features to the voice? Is the vocabulary appropriate for the patient's age? The quality of the grammar allows one to make a reasonable guess about education, if not intelligence. Peculiar slang might indicate something about cultural background or regional origins. What is the affect? Is it the flat, slow, unemotional speech of the depressed patient? Or is it the rapid, pressured speech of a manic patient? How is the language organized? Does this patient speak logically and in full sentences that are responsive to the question, or is he "loose," offering flights of ideas and speaking "word salads" that are hard to follow?

The thoughts underlying speech are also critically important. Does he or she seem to be preoccupied with a particular problem? For example, a paranoid schizophrenic having a full-blown psychotic episode might continually interrupt an interview whenever he heard someone walking down the hall. This observation might guide the interviewer to ask questions about whether the patient had ever experienced phenomena called "Schneiderian first rank symptoms," known after decades of experience to be features of many schizophrenic illnesses. The first rank symptoms include auditory hallucinations, thought manipulation, and thought broadcasting. For example, when trying to assess this diagnostic possibility one might ask a patient, "Do you ever hear voices commenting on things you are doing just as though people were speaking to you? Do you ever feel that someone is putting thoughts into your mind? Do you sometimes get the feeling that everyone knows what you are thinking?"

A patient suffering from schizophrenia might reply that he did hear voices in his head. I distinctly remember one old man who told me that he no longer rode public buses because the passengers near him usually knew what he was thinking. Sometimes they even could enter his mind and change the street corner at which he planned to get off!

On first reading the Schneiderian questions, I just couldn't believe their value. Then, one day I interviewed Jim, a slightly built seventeen-year-old who wound up in the hospital after the police had found him destroying a phone booth with his guitar. His curly brown hair and playful grin lighted up his pale, delicate features. He wore the uniform of a typical New Haven teenager, a T-shirt and blue jeans, and he struck me as a typical adolescent. When I started interviewing Jim, however, his manner seemed inappropriate. He told me where he lived and about his family in a logical way. But, I noticed that he had a curious habit of pointing his index finger at different parts of the room as he spoke.

"What are you doing with your hands?"

"I'm just warming up cold objects with my laser beams," he said.

"Laser beams?"

"Yeah. If you turn your face to the sun and wait quietly you can draw in enough energy to create *laser power!* Then you can share this energy with other things that don't get enough sunlight."

This exchange triggered a long discussion about Jim's world. He believed the sun was the source of all energy, which included forces of *good* and the ability to acquire true *knowledge*. Light of any type was the most precious substance in the world, and its value was determined by its color. White was the greatest, red second, and so forth. The most dreaded thing in the universe was a black hole, which could suck light up and never return it. Although Jim frequently zapped people with his lasers, it was only on command from a *light source* and only to do *good*. (By now I was asking all the Schneiderian questions.) Jim told me that from his hospital window at night he "listened" to the lights on the streets of New Haven.

I concluded the intake interview convinced that Jim was pretty strange, but wondering whether he was merely putting me on. A few more interactions, however, convinced me that he really did have a very tenuous hold on reality. Jim could not sit still in patient-staff meetings. He would speak frequently without raising his hand. He was obviously deeply taken with the notion of "community." He delivered long, convoluted speeches on what constituted the ideal world, reaffirming his hatred of darkness and violence and his love of peace and light. When I asked him about using his guitar to smash a phone booth, he repeatedly said that the phone gave out evil messages, and that a street light had told him to destroy it. When my rotation ended, Jim was just barely functioning in the community, under hefty doses of phenothiazines. He spent his evenings looking out at the thousands of lights that dotted New Haven, waiting for his messages. His prognosis was very grave.

The mental status exam is usually used to determine the orientation, memory, "fund of knowledge," ability to reason abstractly, and judgment skills of the patient. The exam permits an overall assessment of the patient's grounding in reality and some insight into whether the illness is organic or "functional." Orientation is measured to person, place, and time. The physician asks the patient his name, where he is, and the day of the month. Patients suffering from an organic disease such as Alzheimer's may know only their name. Chronically depressed patients who have been in the hospital for months may get no closer to the date than being able to identify the season.

Memory is assessed at two levels: recent and remote. A good way to test recent memory is with serial 7's (or serial 3's if the patient has an extremely limited education). The patient is asked to count back from 100 by subtracting 7 and to continue that operation until he is told to stop. To subtract the patient must "remember" the number from which he is subtracting while he performs the operation. He must also remember to change the number he is "holding" with each subtraction. To test more remote memory the psychiatrist will tell the patient to remember three random words, for example "pencil, lamp, and Broadway." Five minutes later he will interrupt his interview to ask the patient to recall the three items. The error rate on this test is high; normal people often forget one of the three. The memory tests are nonspecific. Poor responses may be a sign of organic disease or a lack of cooperation, or they may merely reflect the patient's stress over the interview. Even psychotic patients can perform well on these tests, so they are helpful in ruling out "organicity."

The fund of knowledge questions permit the examiner to make a crude assessment of the patient's education and intellect. The patient is asked a series of odd questions. Name the last three presidents. What is a telephone? How far is it from Los Angeles to New York City? What does the stomach do? Where is Belgium? Of course the questions can be made as difficult as necessary. Who wrote *Moby Dick*? What causes iron to rust? The answers give some insight into intelligence, attention span, and willingness to cooperate, but they offer little direct insight into a patient's illness.

My favorite questions in the mental status exam were similarities and proverbs. They were intended to judge the higher, cognitive functions of the brain. To test the ability to "see" similarities, we ask the patients to state how paired items are alike. An easy first question might be: "What is the same about a plum and a pear?" to which the answer (which I never heard missed by a person without organic disease) is "fruit." A harder question would be to compare "laughter and tears," both signs of human emotion. I drew a total blank when I was asked the toughest question on the scale: "How are a fly and a tree alike?" They are of course "both living things."

It was actually fun to ask the patients to explain "proverbs." The answers provide some insight into an individual's ability to think abstractly. As with similarities, the examiner usually asks proverbs that are progressively more difficult to answer. A favorite first proverb question is, "What does it mean when I say that people in glass houses should not throw stones?" A typical answer would be: "You

shouldn't criticize others for faults you also may have."
Persons suffering from schizophrenia might answer, "If you
throw stones you will break the glass." Their response is
said to be "concrete," popular psychiatric jargon, suggesting that they have a tenuous hold on reality and are holding
on as best they can. Besides "concreteness," interviewers
also watch for highly personalized answers such as, "I could
get put in jail if I threw stones." Some proverbs are quite
difficult to interpret, especially for those sitting in the
strange new world of a psychiatric unit under the probing
eyes of a shrink. While most patients can explain the
aphorism that "every cloud has a silver lining," very few
can interpret why "the tongue is the enemy of the neck." I
found the silence that usually greeted this proverb to be
ironically appropriate. After all, too much talk may get one
in trouble.

I conducted the mental status exam on about a dozen
patients during my six weeks on the floor. With time I
accepted that it could be used as a screen to help determine whether the patient had a chance to function on the
ward. It was most useful with elderly patients suffering
from senility, patients who drift in and out of reality as their
cortical function waxes and wanes. Months after my psychiatric training ended, I used serial mental status exams to
monitor the return of cognitive function in a patient who
had arrived from a nursing home in a coma from severe
dehydration.

Although the physical environment and the staff nurses
exercised great influence on the "climate" in the therapeutic community, the most important forces were clearly the
patients themselves. In a society of seventeen patients,
most of whom were teenagers, everyone knew each other
well. In a real sense the "state" of the community de-

pended on how the patients got along. A few deadheads or even a single rebellious patient could severely compromise the various group meetings and slow everybody's progress.

Perhaps the best way to illustrate this is to describe the dynamics of the small group with which I worked. Six patients met with Jerry and me twice a week: Pat, Linda, "Sleepy," Bob, Peter, and Juanita. Pat was a "butch"-looking sixteen-year-old who had been forced to have sex with her father and her older brother many times when she was eleven and twelve. She was now a school delinquent and had recently slit her wrists. Linda was a twenty-six-year-old graduate student in history. She was suffering from anorexia nervosa (an eating disorder in which the patient often stops eating completely, and which is sometimes fatal) and had entered the hospital with only sixty-seven pounds on her five-foot four-inch frame. A brilliant student, Linda was a complete recluse and had never had a boyfriend. Sleepy was a sixty-year-old mechanic and an avid CB radio fan with a long history of manic-depressive illness. Prior to this hospitalization he had stopped going to work and had started staying up all night "fixing things" about the house. He had passed several nights taking his refrigerator apart and putting it back together. Now on Lithium, he was no longer "manic." In fact, he denied any illness whatsoever. Bob was the highly intelligent, meticulously mannered seventeen-year-old who was struggling with schizophrenia. Peter, a bearded, overweight, unkempt twenty-four-year-old, had a long history of drug abuse and depression. Before being hospitalized he had spent six months living at home with his mother, smoking dope around the clock and demanding complete care. Before coming to the hospital he had reached the point where he would soil himself rather than go to the toilet. Juanita was a sixteen-year-old Puerto Rican girl who had a long history of promiscuity and drug abuse. She also had made a suicidal "gesture," as the new pink scars on her wrists indicated.

Imagine our small group, six patients, Jerry, and I, locked together in a circle for an hour. The rule was that the patients, not the staff, would do the "work." They would do the talking. I witnessed about a dozen of these sessions, which, despite minor variations, moved in a discernible pattern. After Jerry made some brief administrative announcements a great silence would descend. After several long minutes of restless movements and side-long glances, Bob, easily the most motivated to "get well," would begin the work. He might describe his thoughts that week, repeat a conversation with his father, or ask somebody a question. On a good day he might strike a theme, "getting along with parents," for example, that was important to others in the group and draw some response. Typically, a conversation might last ten minutes before the next long pause.

By quarter past the hour Sleepy was nodding off. His CB "handle," emblazoned in white across his turquoise sweatshirt, was richly deserved. He simply would not stay awake. I never once heard him offer a remark. At various times he attributed this reticence to fatigue, a faulty hearing aid, being overmedicated (he was not), and boredom. Juanita, who had quit junior high school at fourteen, also almost never spoke more than a few words. She seemed unintelligent, had no insights into other patients' problems, and when she spoke at all it was to reiterate her wish to stay away from drugs and men when she "got out." Still under heavy medication that gave her posture a certain rigidity and masked her facial expressions, she sat like an automaton, smoking cigarette after cigarette.

If Sleepy and Juanita were unable to work well in these sessions, Peter was unwilling. His behavior was perfectly predictable. He usually sat quietly, greeting each conversational twist with a contemptuous smirk. About once a week he would openly attack the "therapeutic community," disparaging its goals, denying his own illness, and telling the others that if they were sick, they would never get well here. He obviously intimidated Juanita, who often cried after one of his tirades. Bob was the only one who would respond directly to Peter's bullying. It was obvious that he, always neat and polite, felt utter contempt for Peter's slovenly habits. Unless Jerry intervened, they quickly became entangled in a debate over the value of their therapy that rapidly degenerated to personal attacks. Peter's sole purpose at these meetings was to play the saboteur. He constantly expressed a desire to leave the hospital, yet never signed the "five-day paper" that would guarantee his release.

Pat, newly arrived on the floor and deeply unhappy, could not be coaxed to discuss her own painful past. She was willing to talk to others about their problems, but her participation was fragmentary. Except for Peter, Linda was probably the most self-centered. Wishing only to talk about her "problems," she quickly stopped participating if they were not the subject. Oddly enough she did not consider conflict with her parents, her fear of sexuality, or her life-threatening weight loss to be among those problems. Instead, she spoke constantly about her career goals, totally denying the real issues.

Time and again I left these small group sessions convinced of their futility. Two of the patients, Sleepy and Juanita, had such poor verbal skills that they could barely participate. Linda and Pat could be coaxed into conversation. Peter's sole pleasure was sabotage; he wanted the group to fail. Bob frequently complained that these sessions were useless. When I voiced my concerns to Jerry, he urged me to be patient and search for the little victories. "If Juanita speaks up at all, it's a therapeutic advance," he argued. During my last week on the floor Peter left; his insurance coverage had run out. A new patient entered the group and the dynamics showed signs of improvement.

Just as the success of the small group meetings depended on the conduct of each patient so did the state of the community as a whole. The arrival of a new patient, the departure of an old patient (especially, a "leader"), or even a sudden shift in a person's illness sent ripples throughout this tiny society. Sometimes such changes precipitated a crisis; the various groups would be mired in silence and the community would grind to a halt like some giant, slow-moving freight train out of fuel.

Departures were usually the least disturbing. The staff had at least a week to prepare the community. The strategy was to urge the departing person "to work hard" at talking over his or her hopes and fears about the outside. How well had he prepared his return to reality? Where would she live? What would he do? Who could she turn to for help? There was also a special rule that allowed departing patients and their families to return twice a week (to family meetings) to talk over the problems of transition. The staff had an effective strategy to counter the sense of loss that enveloped the community when a patient departed. The event was turned into a celebration. Every patient was honored with a farewell party, which, in the case of the more popular people, could be quite elaborate. The solarium was decorated with balloons, paper lanterns, and banners. The usual hospital dinners were refused in favor of spaghetti and meatballs made, with great deliberation and lots of disagreements, by the patients in the ward kitchen. It was hilarious to watch six or seven frantic teenagers, all vying to use one electric stove.

Arrivals were always difficult. The patients were extremely sensitive and very perceptive about the impact that a newcomer would have in their society. For example, within a day after she arrived, it was clear that Joanne, a talkative college student with a seductive manner, would climb through the status changes as fast as possible. She was better educated than most of her fellow citizens, and she was a superb flirt, certain to win votes from the men. She immediately recognized the premium placed on "serious" talks among patients, and made a special point of engaging in such encounters all afternoon. Naturally, she could not rise to advisory council without causing some jealousy. When she was elected to the council only ten days after her arrival, the only dissenters were a few of the women in the community.

Mark's arrival was completely different. Mark was a twenty-four-year-old pharmacy student, the son of elderly Polish immigrants, who was suffering from paranoid schizophrenia. About an hour after he came to the floor, I met him and conducted the standard "intake" physical. He was a big, thick-set guy with blazing eyes and an angry look. Quite frankly, he scared me. He was unusually worried about being seen naked. Only after I promised him that he could leave his undershorts on did he consent to the physical examination. He lay back on the table and I approached him cautiously, but when I gently palpated his abdomen he leaped up, shouting at me: "I'm not gay. I'm not gay." I managed to reassure him that my concern was merely to perform a brief exam and that I did not wish to threaten him, but only the most cursory evaluation was possible.

If Mark frightened me, he terrified the patients. He was mercurial; the most innocent remark could make him combative. Bigger than the other patients, he was quick to move in on them, fists clenched, never touching, but threatening them. He pestered the women, grinning lasciviously as he suggested private talks. By his third day on the ward Mark had become an "item of discussion" at

patient-staff meetings. When his name turned up on the
agenda patients' hands flew up around the room. Little
Jim, who was perhaps most terrified of Mark, spoke for
everyone.

"This guy is crazy and he's mean. Everyone's scared of
him. He's wrecking the community. If he doesn't change, I
am taking out a five-day paper."

The five-day paper was the means by which patients
could exercise their legal right to leave the ward despite
the objection of their doctors. It was the ultimate threat
that a patient could pose to the organization of the community and, although frequently made, it was rarely carried
out. After the patients vented their feelings, which in this
case were quite justifiable, the staff tried to explain that
Mark's actions were part of his illness. But nobody, least of
all the fragile young people, could tolerate Mark's combative ways. He behaved like a classic bully.

Two days later, while arguing about who would talk to
Joanne, Mark punched one of the other patients. This act
was unforgivable; he was restricted to his room and placed
on "staff special"—round-the-clock observation, roughly
the equivalent of a jail sentence in society at large. The
community immediately breathed a sigh of relief. With
Mark under house arrest, the solarium and back rooms
were safe again. The community reacted exactly as might
townfolk after the arrest of a mugger who had been terror-
izing old ladies at night. The common link that illness
forged among the patients did not extend to Mark. Despite
the fact that he was one of the most troubled people in the
community (and at times floridly psychotic), nobody attributed his behavior to illness. Mark was still under arrest
when I finished my clerkship.

The most disturbing aspect of life in the therapeutic
community was that the patients were regularly reminded

that, despite every effort made by the staff, some people did not get better. During my stay on the floor a young, acutely psychotic woman named Tanya personified the deepest fears of the others. And with good reason. Tanya's room was a shadow world of terror. Despite extremely heavy medication, her days and night were full of voices that frightened her and put thoughts into her head. She would spend hours rocking back and forth in a fetal position or stalking her room like a caged animal. Some days she could not bear the feeling of being clothed and hardly tolerated a loose bathrobe. Her speech was a high-pitched, repetitive, never-ending plea to go home to her mother. Although she had no desire to converse, she could not stand being alone. Day after day a nurse sat at the door of her room watching over her and trying to talk her back to reality. So taxing was this vigil that the "Tanya shift" changed every hour or two.

Because she was unable to cope with the simple tasks of dressing herself or talking to other people, Tanya rarely left her room, and so the other patients hardly knew her. The rule was that all patients were citizens, so her "progress" was a routine part of the news discussed at community meetings. The patients listened just as we might listen to reports about the condition of a neighbor housebound by illness. Over the weeks, I learned that because of the gravity of her psychosis, Tanya, although "invisible," had a significant influence on the other patients. She was the person who patients compared themselves to when they wished to rationalize the belief that they were not really sick or that they were making progress.

Another reason for the importance of Tanya to the community was that her mother, desperately unhappy about her daughter and overwhelmed with anxiety about the lack of progress, was a faithful participant in family meetings, even though Tanya could not attend. Uneducated, divorced, poor, and suffering from psychiatric problems herself, Tanya's mother would sometimes "take off" on long monologues about the comforts provided by the Bible. The staff, families, and patients would sit in embarrassed silence as she poured out her despair, sometimes punctuated by Tanya's cries drifting down the hall. This family's tragedy coalesced the others in sympathy.

During my fourth week on the floor, Tanya suddenly showed marked improvement. In a few days she became able to dress herself, obey simple instructions, and sit quietly in a group for fifteen minutes. Since she had satisfied these tasks, the staff decided to bring Tanya back, step by step, into the community. She was given permission to attend one meeting a day for thirty minutes. For four consecutive days she managed to do this, sitting quietly, staring blankly ahead, chain smoking cigarettes in imitation of the other women, then leaving when her time was up. Everyone was hopeful, and some of the staff even began to assert privately that Tanya's progress was evidence that the "therapeutic community" worked.

Then disaster struck. One Friday Tanya attended her first patient-staff meeting (at which the entire community assembled). These meetings, which lasted for an hour, were held in the solarium. About thirty people sat on folding chairs and benches in a large "democratic" circle and discussed the business of the society. The assembly was not unlike a town meeting in Vermont. The energy level at patient-staff hour was usually very high, and the staff knew it was taking a risk by allowing Tanya to attend. Although she sat between two of the floor nurses, who were trying to keep her calm, Tanya's circuits were quickly overloaded. Within minutes she was breaking the rules, standing up, walking a few steps into the center of the room and then going to a new seat, and talking, without being recognized, about topics unrelated to the business at hand. Suddenly, she was crying, begging to leave the room. The nurse next to her could not calm her, and Tanya slumped to the floor. We had to drag her from the center of the meeting amidst stunned silence.

This setback was especially ominous because Tanya's insurance coverage was due to expire in ten days. There seemed to be hardly any chance that she would recover in time to be discharged to her mother's care. In fact, she continued to regress. She left in a hail of screams by ambulance for the large state institution known as "Hell" among the patients. This was the place where nobody got better. Tanya's was the most dreaded disposition of all.

Life on the tenth floor had its humorous moments, too. One of the funniest was when I chaperoned the weekly trip to the local YMCA for volleyball. This highly organized and greatly prized outing was a breath of freedom for the patients. Promptly at 2:30 twelve patients dressed in sweatshirts, shorts, and an odd variety of sneakers lined up with me at the ward door. A buzzer sounded, the door opened, and we took a special transport elevator to the lobby. In front of the hospital, a yellow school bus was waiting to take us on a half-mile ride to the gym. Once they were on the bus a sense of exhilaration swept through the patients—at least those who were not deeply depressed or heavily medicated. Sherry, a voluptuous fifteen-year-old with a blaring radio, was dancing in the aisle, while the rest were hanging out the windows and chattering about the sights as though on the first leg of a two-week package tour of Italy. After surveying the scene, Bob, who was sitting next to me, grinned widely as he said, "We're all Bozos on this bus."

One of the gyms was reserved for us, and the volleyball net was already set up. Picking up sides required more deliberation than most of the kids could muster, so I chose the teams. We were just about to play when loud rock 'n' roll burst from the next gym. Sherry squealed and raced off, followed more slowly by a couple of others. They flung the door open. The adjoining gym was filled with about thirty black kids on roller skates. From the doorway we watched them race around the gym, flawlessly executing the fancy steps of roller-disco. Sherry rushed to grab some free skates. Visions of broken ankles and elbows filled my mind. It took my sternest voice and firmest grip to drag her back to volleyball. She spent the rest of the hour in center court boogeying to the sounds from next door.

Have you ever tried to organize twelve adolescents with psychiatric illness to play volleyball? Forget the rules about rotating positions, serving within boundary markers, or hitting the ball only three times before returning it. Don't try to keep score. In our game the object of serving was to determine how far one could hit the ball. Since the gym was ancient and quite small, most serves caromed off the ceiling. Fortunately, we only cracked one window pane. I tried for a few minutes to organize some team spirit and play competitively, but I quickly returned to reality. At least we could get some exercise.

My team was virtually assured of scoring points if only the server could put the ball over the net and in bounds. This was because the opposition's center court was occupied by that team's worst player—who refused to rotate positions. Richard, a patient with chronic schizophrenia, was heavily medicated and rarely moved faster than a slow shuffle. After about eight tries Sherry finally made a good serve, a low drive that just cleared the middle of the net, going right at Richard. I couldn't believe my eyes. He stared at the ball, watching it approach, and did not move an inch. It struck him full in the face, bouncing high to his left where Bob deftly returned it for a point. All the players congratulated Richard on a beautiful assist! Despite the red circle on his cheek, Richard was beaming, apparently uninjured and proud of his play. Thus the game continued, out of bounds serves alternating with blows to chins and heads. In about fifteen minutes everybody was exhausted and I called a halt. Depending on their medications, the patients either promptly curled up to rest on the floor mats or raced to watch the roller-disco. A few minutes later it was time to return to the bus.

One "drawback" to taking my clerkship in the therapeutic community was that most patients were not acutely ill. They came to our ward only after hospitalization in another unit that specialized in neuropsychiatric evaluation. It was there that they started on medications and calmed down. Thus, I really appreciated the three nights I spent with a resident working in the emergency room (ER). All the patients we saw there were acutely ill. The ER psychiatric resident hung out in a little room that reminded me of a real estate office—a couple of desks, a coffee table, an arm chair, and a lot of ash trays. Some nights there would be no patients; other nights all hell would break loose. If just one patient was "genuinely" ill, the task of assessing and placing him in a world where it was very tough to find open "psychiatric beds" could take most of the night.

On my first two nights in the ER, things were boringly quiet, but on my last night I saw two dramatically ill patients. The first was the most bizarrely acting person I have ever seen, and the second probably depressed me more than had any other patient. Jerry and I were sitting in the "real-estate office," hunched over coffee when we got called to the "detox" room, where the more belligerent alcoholics were strapped into beds to sleep it off. Usually the psychiatric resident did not get involved in their management. Over the phone the nurse told Jerry that an ambulance had brought in a "real wild man" who was screaming about his restraints. "Now's your chance to try an acute exam," said Jerry, and off I went.

His name was Barry Washington. He was a tall, muscu-

lar black man, about twenty-two years old, who the police
told me they had brought in at the request of his mother. I
found him lying with a sheet wrapped around his head and
his arms and legs bound by thick leather straps to the edge
of the bed. According to his mother, who stood tearfully in
the doorway, for the last two days Barry had been extremely agitated. He had been breaking plates and furniture and spent hours in his room doing vigorous calisthen-
ics. Realizing that she would be a much better source of
information than Barry, I found a corner for us to talk
privately.

Although nothing like this had ever happened before,
Barry's world had been deteriorating for nearly three
years. After a normal life as an average student in high
school, he had gone off to a small college on a basketball
scholarship. He had flunked out after one semester. The
following year another attempt at another college lasted
only a few weeks. He enlisted in the Air Force and did well
for a year before he was suddenly discharged due to
"erratic behavior." His mother had no knowledge about the
specifics of this period. After returning home, he had
gotten his first steady job as a night watchman and had
managed to hang on to it. But eighteen months ago he had
joined a fringe religious group, popular among ex-acid
heads, called "Holiness." He went to meetings several
times a week and was very devout. He had told his mother
that he had "connected" with God. Last week Barry had
suddenly quit his job and moved home with his mother.
He spent hours talking to people who were not present and
behaving in a totally disruptive way. His mother was
mystified, but she was also tired of putting up with him.
After he had started throwing bottles against the kitchen
wall and singing gospel songs, she called the police. I
thanked her for this information, tried to reassure her, and
marched back into the room.

He was still wrapped in the sheet as though it were a

shroud. I tapped on his bed rail, introduced myself, and asked if we could talk. Slowly, he drew the sheet down, revealing a handsome, short-haired black man with a wild look in his eyes. To my surprise, he was willing to talk.

"How are you feeling?" I asked.

The response came like machine gun fire. I could not believe anybody could talk that quickly. "I am feeling very, very good. I eat right, stay fit, and keep close to God."

"How do you stay close to Him?"

"I have a partnership with God. We speak regularly. I know what He looks like. He guides me."

I asked next how his daily life was going. His demeanor suddenly changed, and a very suspicious look crept over him.

"Too many people know where I live, so I moved."

"What do you do for fun? Do you still play basketball?"

"I'm pro material," he exclaimed, "but I don't want all that traveling."

I launched into a formal mental status exam, but I didn't get far. He did know where he was and how he got there, but he refused to do calculations, explain proverbs, or perform any of the other tests.

"Only if you untie me," was his stock response.

"I can't do that, Barry. You are in restraints because you have been doing dangerous things."

He hassled with me for another minute, and then he dove back under the sheets to silence. A few minutes later without ever having met Jerry, Barry was bundled back into an ambulance. Given that he was a vet and that private psychiatric beds were rare, we had turfed him to the local VA hospital.

I was just getting ready to head home when our next patient arrived. She was a small, quiet black woman with shabby clothes, flat affect, and downcast eyes. Her name was Mollie, she was twenty-seven, and she came to the ER asking to be admitted to the Connecticut Mental Health

Center "for a rest." After making this announcement to us, she sat down on the couch as though the matter were decided and all that remained was the paperwork. Jerry slowly and carefully began to question her. She lived in a cold-water flat with her five-year-old son; her income was partly from welfare benefits and partly from prostitution. She had family in the neighborhood. She appeared depressed, but she was well oriented and her cognition was clearly intact. After about an hour of questioning, Jerry told her that she did not need to be admitted to the hospital. He advised her to go home to her son, who was sleeping in the apartment alone, and return in the morning if she felt the need to talk with a psychiatrist.

Her answer knocked my socks off.

"If you don't admit me," she said slowly and deliberately, "I'll go home and kill my son and myself with gas."

There was a long pause. Jerry excused himself, and we left the room. He was furious. "She has got us by the balls. She knows the system better than I do. I can't turn away a suicide or homicide threat. It's too big a risk."

His fury was spent in five minutes. There was a lot to do. First we called the police to go and pick up her son. We would have to place him temporarily in a foster home. Then we began the long process of admitting her.

The police arrived an hour later. The little boy was dressed in red sneakers, summer clothes, and a baseball hat. Although it was below freezing, he had no coat. The police had found him alone in an unlocked apartment. They had also managed to locate his fifteen-year-old cousin, who came along to help. Mollie was sitting alone in the little side room, smoking a cigarette. After I told her that her son had arrived, she smiled faintly but made no move to go to him. I went back to the little boy and asked him if he wanted to visit his mother. He looked solemnly at me and said simply, "No." I felt overwhelming sadness for him and all the lousy breaks he was getting. How did a kid like this have a chance to enjoy life? What was it like to never feel loved? How could his mother act like that? Could she really be that sick? I wanted to feel sympathy for her, but I hated her because of what she was doing to her son.

About an hour later the paperwork was done, and Jerry gave me the job of escorting Mollie to the mental health center. A curious warren of underground tunnels connects the hospital buildings. They are an endless array of low-ceilinged vaults that are crisscrossed by pipes, wires, and heating vents and decorated with years of medical grafitti. Our steps echoed as we made the quarter-mile trip. It was like the setting of a murder mystery. I deliberately walked half a step behind Mollie, wondering all the way how disturbed she really was. To my surprise when we arrived on the ward the nurse greeted her by name. After Mollie had been put into bed, I asked the nurse how she knew her new patient.

"Oh, she pulls this bullshit every December. She's a sociopath all right, but she's crazy like a fox. She can't afford a trip to Miami so she takes her winter vacation here. I just pity her son."

The most that a medical student can accomplish during a six-week tour of duty on a psychiatric floor is to develop a feel for the mystery of mental illness and the ways in which doctors and nurses try to help their patients. Unlike the world of internal medicine, one cannot note a patient's physical findings and combine them with an array of laboratory values to reach a clear-cut diagnosis and choose a therapeutic course. The most sophisticated analysis of the body will usually not prove that a psychiatric patient may be desperately ill. Psychiatrists face the toughest diagnostic challenges in medicine. Each day they must try to decide where a patient "fits" in the huge spectrum of psychic disturbances, which nonpsychiatrists lump under the phrase "mental illness." In a single afternoon the psychiatrist may see an adolescent trying to cope with the "normal" stresses of his age and offer therapy to a man who has been imprisoned by schizophrenia for twenty years. The doctor knows that the adolescent will probably rebound after short-term psychotherapy; the chronic schizophrenic faces a much bleaker future.

Most of us have developed a remarkable ability to deal with life's pressures. But the intensity of those pressures can increase at any time, and, just as everyone has a unique threshhold to physical illness, we all vary in our ability to cope with psychic stress. Fortunately, psychiatry helps most people deal with the monsters of rage, guilt, sadness, fear, and uncertainty that prowl restlessly inside the mind. Armed with psychotherapeutic skills, medicines, and infinite patience, a good psychiatrist usually can help restore the mysterious coping mechanisms. The vast majority of patients who seek psychiatric care never require hospitalization or else spend relatively short sojourns in therapeutic communities.

The small percentage of patients who are burdened with profound mental distress face a vastly different prognosis. I had come to the clerkship full of textbook knowledge about how phenothiazines and tricyclics had revolutionized the care of such individuals. True, many acutely psychotic people, cut adrift from reality in a sea of madness, benefit tremendously from drug therapy. The medicines pull them back toward shore, to within reach of the therapeutic community. Neither medicines nor milieus cure the patients who lapse into chronic illnesses. Drugs may subdue florid madness, but they do not offer a straight road back to a normal life.

I did not see a "cure" in my six weeks on psychiatry. Those who left the floor "well" had not come in with serious illness. They were mostly adolescents who had decompensated under stress, and who were shunted into the system due to the lack of a normal "support" structure at home. Most people who left the floor did so because their insurance had run out. They usually returned to a world that tolerated them fairly well. For the few who were profoundly ill, the last "paid" day was indeed black: Their next home would be a state facility, a world with fewer environmental comforts and a much grimmer psychic climate.

I finished the psychiatric clerkship with mixed emotions. During my six weeks in the therapeutic community, I had come to believe all too well in the reality of mental illness. Heretofore I had imagined that psychiatrists spent their hours listening to upper-class people rant about their personal discontents, their sexual frustrations, and their bruised egos. Now I knew that psychiatrists helped to heal real hurts. Especially toward those men and women who work at "inpatient" facilities, I will always feel deep admiration. They face a career marked by therapeutic failures that match those faced by neurosurgeons and oncologists.

Chapter 7

MRS. LANDI

The clinical year is rich in intimacy. Every physician remembers a few special faces from the first months in which he or she learned to care for patients. If one patient made me a physician, it was a woman I met on a gray morning early in January. The grueling clerkship year was more than half over, and I was starting my second "medical clerkship." This six-week period was reputed to be the pinnacle of the third year. It was here that a student was supposed to become most involved in patient care and be most closely watched by the residents and attending faculty members.

By Monday evening I realized that this emergence as a player on the team was not going to happen. The hospital floor where most of our patients would stay had been closed over the Christmas holidays. It had reopened just two days before, and only four patients were on the twenty-four-bed floor. To exacerbate matters further, the medical team was as overpopulated as the patient census was low. On that first Monday morning there gathered together two residents, two interns, two subinterns, and four medical students. A team of ten had assembled to care for a total of eight patients—four on the tenth floor and four housed elsewhere.

The senior resident, Dick Sauer, perhaps the most competent and compassionate house officer I met in medical school, reassured the students that the census would grow rapidly during the next two weeks. Nevertheless, having spent the better part of a year waiting to get more involved, the four of us took this news with a grain of salt. My concerns grew when I heard that both subinterns were fourth-year students from other medical schools and had come here to help their chances of being chosen as interns by Yale for the coming year. They both seemed eager to acquire a large patient load as quickly as possible. Because they were still trying to master the procedures that we were just learning—spinal taps, paracentesis—and because this would be their first chance "to run" the cases, I guessed that third-year students would not get very deeply involved with their patients.

After we had finished rounds on the tenth floor the team trooped downstairs to the seventh floor to visit the rest of our patients. As we huddled outside her door, the junior resident, a brilliant young woman, told us about Mrs. Landi.

"This seventy-nine-year-old, married Italian lady was admitted to this hospital for the first time three days ago to work up an anemia that was discovered by her private physician. Her story begins ten days ago when she saw her doctor with complaints of increasing fatigue over the last two weeks and easy bruising. He obtained a hematocrit of 28, and he decided to admit her for an anemia workup.

"Her physical exam was unremarkable except for a grade two over six systolic ejection murmur heard best at the lower left sternal border, large bruises over her forearms and thighs, and moderate arthritic changes in her hands. Her EKG and chest x-ray were normal as were her other admission lab tests. A peripheral blood smear done on her first day here contained many erythroid precursors and was highly suggestive of Di Guglielmo's disease. The hematologist to whom she was referred has performed a bone marrow biopsy, which confirmed the diagnosis.

"Plans for her are uncertain. The hematologist is talking the case over with Mrs. Landi's family and they will decide whether to send her home or put her on the latest protocol. OK, let's go in and say hello."

As we crowded into the small room I was still uncertain as to just what was wrong with this lady, but the resident's tone of voice had made it clear that Mrs. Landi was in big trouble. After making a mental note to read up on Di Guglielmo's disease, which I remembered vaguely as a type of leukemia, I turned to the patient's bed. As I surveyed the room I had to smile. It was as though we were grandchildren visiting grandmother on her birthday. Mrs. Landi sat propped up in bed, an empty breakfast tray across her lap. She was wrapped in a shocking pink sweater and a big smile. She greeted us each in turn as we were introduced and asked us how *we* were feeling. Her eyes were bright and dancing and she seemed happy.

"Well, Mrs. Landi," said the resident, "today's the day we decide whether to give you the special medicines for the tired blood."

"Good! Good! Whatever Dr. Shaw and my boys think is best."

"Any questions for us Mrs. Landi?"

"No."

"OK. Have a nice day."

And we marched out.

I was puzzled. Although still a tyro, I knew that the phrase "latest protocol" was ominous. It usually meant that the patient was about to be hit with three or more very potent drugs—in the hope that they would somehow stop a cancer that was rampaging through the body. It often meant terrible side effects: pain, vomiting, hair loss. It also meant infection because these drugs crippled the body's natural defenses, and it could mean death. Yet, when we had visited her, Mrs. Landi had been smiling and happy. Indeed, she had been in higher spirits than the house staff. There could be only one conclusion: She was not yet aware of her illness.

That night I pulled Harrison's *Principles of Internal Medicine* (the medical student's bible) off my shelf, and read the paragraph or two devoted to Di Guglielmo's disease. I learned that this was the eponym for a rare form of leukemia involving the precursors from which red blood cells are made. It was characterized by bizarre immature red blood cells and a hyperactive bone marrow (the place where blood is made). No one had reported good success in treating persons with this illness, and it was considered to be a rapidly fatal disease. Why, I wondered, would doctors or the family want to put a patient her age on a devastating group of drugs if she had almost no chance of surviving anyway? Did the patient and the family understand what they were getting into?

At rounds the next day I learned that the patient census had only increased by two. As I would not be on call until Thursday, I decided to ask Alfred Madison, the subintern who had been assigned to care for Mrs. Landi, if I could also follow her case. He agreed and I decided to pay her a visit that afternoon.

Until I started medical school I had imagined *death* as a powerful but distant enemy who preyed on the weak and the elderly but had little chance to grab healthy young men. Having spent nearly six months on clinical rotations, I now perceived death as a less remote figure. Now, it was an icon, carved for me by Bergman in his movie *The Seventh Seal*. I imagined death as a brilliant and relentless foe who never lost but could be tricked for a time and delayed. He and Mrs. Landi had reached end-game, and she was in check. There was no chance to avoid mate, but could we develop a defense that would allow her one more summer with her grandchildren? And what would the defense cost her? I thought about this all morning.

At one o'clock I was sitting alone in the hospital cafeteria, ignoring my plate and thinking of my grandmother, the only grandparent I had ever knowm, who had died of cancer ten years ago. I was remembering the pain I had felt that this wonderful, strong woman should waste away to nothing as cancer devoured her bowels. And I was remembering my guilt. Five years had elapsed from the diagnosis and first operation until her death. The last two years had been relentless wasting—*cachexia* was the word I now used. She had lost nearly half her body weight but held onto her spirits until the end. Those five years had been vigorous, happy, carefree, college years for me. Though I loved her dearly, I had offered very little of myself to her. A few visits and an occasional letter were all that I had mustered for a woman who had helped to raise me.

The third year of medical school was more than half over. I had learned a great deal, but I was still a novice. I had seen many patients but had remained on the periphery of their care. Was it not time for me to embrace a patient, to confront suffering and dying as closely as a healthy person can? I found myself taking a vow: As long as she did not object, I would visit Mrs. Landi every day that she stayed in the hospital. I would get to know her as a person, and I would give her whatever comfort and solace that I could. If some grand ledger was kept in the Universe, perhaps I could make up for the debt I owed my grandmother. Little did I realize that I was the one who was going to receive the gift.

Before going in to visit Mrs. Landi, I stopped at the nursing station to reread her records. There I found Dr. John Huxley, a pathologist who was especially expert in the diagnosis of leukemias and lymphomas, putting a note in the chart. I politely accosted him.

"Dr. Huxley, would you explain to me what this erythroid leukemia means for Mrs. Landi? Does that new protocol offer her some hope?"

The trace of a light, sad smile played across his face as Huxley briefly told me that if Mrs. Landi was not treated with the anticancer agents, she would probably die at home within two weeks from a massive internal hemorrhage.

"But, if she does go on the protocol," he said, "she will probably die of a massive infection in the hospital within the next two months. Either way, she's a dead duck."

After Dr. Huxley left, I carefully reread the chart to see whether any doctor had noted that Mrs. Landi understood the gravity of her illness. I learned that she was now under the care of three physicians who specialized in hematology and oncology (cancer). Apparently, one of them had talked the situation over with her three sons, and they had asked him to place their mother on a course of chemotherapy that would begin the next day. What role, I wondered, had Mrs. Landi played in this decision? For that matter, what was her perception of her illness? Did I have any right to raise the subject with her?

Usually, I had a reason, some unpleasant task like drawing blood or doing a rectal exam, for knocking on a patient's door. Then my knock was more or less perfunctory, for I was there on business that could not be denied. But this visit had no medical purpose. So after knocking I waited until a gentle voice beckoned me to come in. She was sitting in an armchair watching one of the soap operas that propel many hospital patients through long, boring afternoons. The smile on her face put me at ease; I felt right away that I was a welcome diversion from the television. I had decided to be as honest as I could.

"Mrs. Landi, my name is Philip Reilly. I am a third-year

medical student working with the doctors who are caring for you. I thought it would be nice for us to get to know each other, if you don't mind."

"Sure, sure. Come in—sit down. What do you want to know?"

Thus began one of the most intimate relationships I have ever known. There were, of course, the required preliminaries, the questions that patients expect doctors to ask. She gave me the medical history that I had been taught to take, and then she told me the bare facts that we use to outline the social and family histories of our patients. Her name was Ada. She had been born the last child of a big family in Italy. When still an adolescent she had married a man who took her away from her family to America. To her, hospitals were places where you had your babies. She had been healthy her whole life, except for one time. During the summertime, maybe in 1936 or 1937, she had lots of belly-pain after eating. In the fall of that year, "they" had taken out her gallbladder. A few years ago she had gotten "the sugar" (diabetes). She was nearly blind in her left eye. She had arthritis in her hands and shoulders, but she still did laundry and cooked.

She had been married for sixty-one years. Her eighty-two-year-old husband, although weakened by a stroke, still got about the house. She had given birth to three sons and one daughter. The saddest time in her life was the winter her little girl, eleven years old, died of kidney failure at the Grace-New Haven Hospital. "The doctors could do nothing," she said. It had been forty-five years, but she weeped as she told me. Her three sons were grown men in their forties, all of whom lived near New Haven.

I encouraged her to talk more about her family and her early years in America. She told her simple story in a delightful way, and before we knew it an hour had passed, and we were feeling at ease with each other. She was a gentle soul, uneducated, whose entire life had centered on her home and family. She was an energetic lady, who after only three days in the hospital was restless to get back to her homemaking chores. She was also a faithful person—"a good Catholic," as she put it. And next to her faith in God and her family, she placed much faith in physicians. It was already clear, before I asked, that she had not questioned her doctors about her illness. When she had been told to pack a bag and come to the hospital she had obeyed.

By now I wanted very much to know what she understood about her illness. I put the question as directly as possible.

"Mrs. Landi, what is wrong with you?"

A dark shadow flitted across her face. She glanced up at me, slowly shrugging her shoulders, with a look of confusion and fear.

"Tired blood."

I waited, but those two words were all she could muster.

"So you know about the special medicines you will start getting tomorrow?"

"No," she said, "explain to me, please."

That was a question that I was not prepared to answer. I had not read the protocol. Suddenly, I was afraid. If I started talking about chemotherapy, I might mislead her or irritate her private physicians, whom I had not even met. I had vowed to be as honest with Mrs. Landi as I could. But all the invisible rules of the medical pecking order and my own lack of self-confidence now welled up in me. She was not "my" patient, and I knew next to nothing about her disease or the treatment planned for her. What right did I have to speak. On the other hand I knew that, despite my lack of expertise, it was true that Mrs. Landi was about to embark on a painful course with only a slim chance for cure. I took a middle ground.

"It's not just that your blood is tired, Mrs. Landi. Some

of the blood is bad; it is not being made right. The medicines will be used to kill the cells that make the bad blood. Then, maybe your body will make good blood."

I paused, wondering what to say about the horrible side effects that might come with the treatment. How do you tell someone she is about to be tortured? I did not have the strength to say what was in my heart. I could not say, "Mrs. Landi, you don't know it yet, but you have a terrible disease that will kill you, no matter what anybody here does. Don't let them treat you. Just go home." Instead, like so many doctors before me, I concocted my own diluted version of the truth.

"These medicines are very powerful. While they are killing the bad cells, they also kill good cells in your body. You will get sick to your stomach, and some of your hair will fall out. Your body will not work as well in fighting germs, so you may get an infection. But in time the good cells should grow back and you will feel better."

I felt like a liar. How could Mrs. Landi know the horror that lurked in my subtle choice of verbs? If the good cells that "should" grow back did not, she would die of massive infection. But I knew it did not really matter. The look on her face told me that she had not understood me. I decided to retreat.

"Do you have any questions for me?"

This was the usual way that doctors ended visits with patients. Her response startled me. She reached out and grasped my hand. Her voice and eyes were pleading, and her grip was iron.

"Tell me true, Doctor Reilly, how long do I gotta stay here?"

She wanted a number so badly. Four days, ten days; anything, as long as she could start the countdown. My words felt so empty.

"I am sorry, Mrs. Landi, I just don't know. You'll have to ask your regular doctors. See you tomorrow, OK?"

It was an hour or so later that Al, the subintern who was caring for Mrs. Landi, asked me to run a typical medical student errand. Would I go across the street to Dr. Handlin's office and pick up a copy of the protocol. For once I agreed without resenting this kind of busy work. What I retrieved was a lengthy, intricate plan for treating erythroleukemia with three powerful anticancer agents. Although the inch-thick document weighed heavy in my hand, its message was quite simple. These drugs would be used to destroy almost completely her hematopoietic (blood-making) system. She would be given whole blood, platelets, and leukocytes to keep her alive during the fourteen days that would elapse between giving the poisons and the recovery of her bone marrow, hopefully in "remission." The goal was to kill all of the cancer cells without killing all of the normal blood-making cells. What were her chances? No one knew, but the protocol writers guessed that patients would have about a 20 percent chance of going into remission. Of those in remission, one-half could expect the disease to reappear within six months. It would then proceed rapidly on its fatal course. Even under the best of circumstances the odds were bad.

At rounds the next morning I learned that Mrs. Landi had started her seven-day course of chemotherapy. A simple sign taped to her door proclaimed, "Mask and Glove Precautions." By wearing gloves and masks we would lessen the shower of germs that we scattered on her each day. Actually, this rule of "reverse isolation" (protecting the patient from the environment) worked mainly by discouraging people from entering the room at all unless they had a specific chore to do. Mrs. Landi would be spending a lot of time alone. How badly, I wondered, would her spirits flag? Given the crudity of this isolation technique, was the gain worth the price? I realized that my daily visits would become all the more important to her.

The next meeting went surprisingly well. Despite the

discomfort of an intravenous line (through which she got her medicines and transfusions) and her confusion about the odd hours at which interns were giving her medicines, Mrs. Landi acted for all the world like a healthy grandmother. My days generally quieted down after "x-ray conference" at 3:30, so I spent the late afternoon in her room, the two of us chatting and watching the pale winter sun set over West Rock.

She did not understand the immense potency of the chemicals that were dripping into her veins, so she could not rejoice (as I did silently) that she was experiencing few discomforting side effects. Instead, still not realizing that her body was held hostage by cancer, she fretted each day about when she could go home. A certain litany developed to the time that we spent together. I would ask after her health, and she would say that she felt fine and could not understand why she was already in the hospital for over a week. I would repeat my half-truths about her illness and the medicines. Then I would try to divert her to other thoughts.

Often I would persuade her to tell me stories of her childhood in Italy. They were simple, but rich and palpable.

"When I was a little girl we were very poor, but I was happy. My parents called me 'the little bird' because I was always singing. I usually sang lullabies to make the babies sleep. In the village we would have dances at night, and I could dance for hours without getting tired at all. I would only stop when my Papa took me home."

One afternoon Mrs. Landi told me a sad story that I will always remember, so heavy is it with irony. It was about 1912; automobiles were still so rare in her part of Italy that weeks would go by before the next one was seen driving along the narrow dirt road through the village. Her home faced onto the road, and often the little children would play on the road's edge while the older children did chores. One day her little brother, deaf since birth, was struck and killed by the only automobile to drive down that road in months. "Surely, God must have wanted him," she said.

At rounds each day, Al reported on Mrs. Landi's management. Because of the mask and glove precautions, several of the medical students and one of the interns on our team had never even seen her. For them, she was a mathematical function, a life known only by a series of numbers that traced the work done by our chemicals. We could not know if we were wiping out her cancer, but as her white cell count fell ever lower—from 9800 to 6400 to 2100 to 1100 to 325 to 25 to 10—we knew we were killing the cells among which the cancer hid. Just as we wanted the white blood cell count to disappear, we could not let the platelets (which keep us from bleeding to death at the slightest trauma) fall too low. Thus the talk at Mrs. Landi's door focused on the esoterica of platelet survival curves. Would the five units of platelets that she had been given the night before raise her count above the critical 50,000 mark—the safety zone, above which bleeding should not be a problem? It did.

The days crawled by; the chemotherapy ran its course. Ten days after we had started her on the protocol, we took a second sample of bone marrow from Mrs. Landi's hip. The pathologist would "read" this tissue and pronounce judgment. Three days later word came; The bone marrow sample showed no evidence of leukemia. She was in remission! I felt a great sense of hope. Maybe Mrs. Landi really would get out of here soon. But I noticed that Bill Keller, the junior resident on the team, was unimpressed with the news. As we walked down the corridor, I asked why. He shook his head. "They always die of pneumonia," was all he said.

But by late afternoon Bill's somber prophecy had faded

to a vague threat. Before knocking, I pulled down the clipboard from its rack by Mrs. Landi's door and glanced over her temperature charts. The nurses took her temperature three times a day. Because we had devastated her white blood cells (these cells are the soldiers in the trenches who fight invading bacteria in hand-to-hand combat), Mrs. Landi was extremely vulnerable. A rising temperature would signal the invasion and trigger a massive counterattack with antibiotics. She had been in the hospital—a building riddled with germs—for fifteen days, but her temperature had held steady at 98.6, as it was today. If we could ward off infection for another week, her white blood count would begin climbing back to normal, and she would be able to go home.

It was a special day. After putting on a gown and mask, I strode into the room with a smile in my eyes. She sat beaming in her armchair, surrounded by her three sons. A few minutes earlier her private physician had told everyone the good news about the bone marrow biopsy. After chatting with her "boys," who profusely thanked me for the hours spent at their mother's bed, I turned to go. Ray, the oldest, took my arm.

"Doc, could we ask you a few questions?"

It was at moments like this that I realized how uneasy I was in my ignorance and how I disliked my perch on the bottom rung of the medical ladder. Should I tell these three men, who clearly thought that I played a crucial role in caring for their mother, that in fact I had never been involved in caring for a person with leukemia until I met her, that all I really did was visit her for a bit each day because I hated to think of her sitting alone in her room, restless and scared, that I was not a doctor? Again, I compromised.

"Well, Mr. Landi, I still have a lot to learn, but I'll try to answer your questions."

A flood gate was opened. From the obvious, "When can

she go home?" which I could not answer, we progressed to ever more difficult topics: What is leukemia? What did the medicines do? Will she have to take them again? Does this mean she is cured? Although I fielded each question, I was pained at the vague and noncommittal words with which I framed my answers. The sentences were horrible. They sounded like the slippery words of some smart lawyer testifying before a senate subcommittee. In the final analysis I was not saying anything. But no sign of dissatisfaction appeared on their faces. At last they had found someone in medicine to whom they could talk with relative ease. In fact I was doing just what good nurses do countless times. After a doctor gives an accurate, but too technical, explanation and leaves, the patient turns to a nurse and asks, "What does all that mean?" And she, despite her limited store of pathophysiological facts, may do a better job of informing him.

The very next day, Mrs. Landi's sixteenth day in the hospital, disaster, with its wonderfully theatrical sense of timing, struck. At six o'clock in the morning she spiked a temperature to 101.6. Because Mrs. Landi was a "protocol" patient, the treatment was automatic. Two weeks earlier she had (without the slightest understanding) signed a form consenting both to the chemotherapy that she had been given and to receive a special regimen of antibiotics if she came down with a fever. Although it was now nearly eight o'clock, no one had yet worked up her fever. The intern on call had been busy with another patient, and Al was himself in bed with the flu. At rounds Bill was visibly upset. In immunosuppressed patients a few hours delay in giving antibiotics can reduce their chances of surviving a bacterial infection. He ordered another intern and me to care for Mrs. Landi until Al was back on his feet. I was told to "break" rounds and do the fever workup now.

The purpose of a fever workup is to find out what kind of bug has invaded the body, where it is hiding, and which antibiotics will kill it. The protocol that guided our management of Mrs. Landi required an unusually detailed workup. Using sterile techniques I would have to draw blood from three separate places, obtain a urine sample by placing a catheter in her bladder, obtain a chest x-ray, get sputum from as far down in her throat as possible, and swab her rectum. I would immediately send these secretions off for "C and S" (culture and sensitivity) to find out what kind of bacterium was growing and which drug could kill it.

I had done dozens of fever workups during the past few months. Although it sometimes took the skill of a wizard to draw blood from the gnarled veins of elderly patients, I felt technically proficient. Something else was troubling me. In two weeks I had become very close to Mrs. Landi, but I had had little to do with her physical care. Suddenly, I would be sticking her with needles, poking her belly, examining her rectum, and hurting her arthritic shoulders as I turned her about in bed. In befriending her I had erected the kind of emotional barrier that makes family members embarrassed to see each other naked. Now I had to breach them. Would she also feel uncomfortable? What should I say?

The concern in my eyes spoiled her smile as I walked into her room. A visit at eight o'clock in the morning was an obvious change in our routine.

"Mrs. Landi, how are you feeling today?"

"Not so good. I have a cough."

"The nurses tell me that you have a temperature, dear. Do you remember how I told you that we must be very careful if you get a temperature, because your defenses are weak? Well, I have to do some tests now to find out if you have an infection, OK? But, first, we'll just do a quick exam to see if you have any pain any place."

She nodded her assent.

First the head. Her skin was moist and warm, but she was not sweating profusely. Her throat was red, but there was no sign of bacterial exudate. Her neck was supple and her lymph nodes were not enlarged. Now the heart and lungs. "Could you lean forward, dear?" I hunched over her, unsnapped the clips to her johnny-coat and zigzagged my stethoscope across her back. The breath sounds were quiet and regular, until I reached the lower right side. There in an area the size of my palm I could hear with each breath a crackling sound like cellophane paper being crumpled. A temperature, a new cough, and rales in the right lung were strongly suggestive of pneumonia. Bill's words flashed through my mind. Was this the beginning of the end? I prodded the four quadrants of her abdomen. No pain there. Gently, remembering that her arthritis was worse on her left shoulder, I turned her on her right side and lifted the johnny-coat to expose her back and buttocks and legs. Her lower back was discolored by a huge purple-blue bruise, as though she had fallen badly. This was one of the consequences of low platelets. Her buttocks, too, were mottled with blood. I pulled them apart to inspect her anus. A small, nasty perianal ulcer, one of the inevitable results of a long time on one's backside, had developed. This was an obvious track for invading bacteria. With a sterile swab I swept the ulcer crater and popped the specimen into a culture tube.

The physical exam completed, I worked quickly to get the bloods drawn; the nurses would do the rest. So far we had not talked much. Now came the tough part.

"Ada, we're going to have to start giving you some new medicines this morning. They are to protect you from infection and you'll be getting them through your IV line for the next ten days." (Such was the protocol.) Her face fell like a stone. Only the night before she had been planning to return home. She had entered the hospital, not knowing what was wrong, expecting to stay two or three days. Instead, she had been cooped up in a little room for sixteen days, and I had just added ten to the sentence.

She clutched my hand and pulled me to the bedside. It had finally dawned that things were more serious than anyone had ever let on.

"Tell me the truth, please. Am I going to get better?"

It is so much easier to lie. I just could not tell her what it meant to get a pneumonia when the white count was less than 100, when the lungs were fertile fields for bacteria. I took the easy way.

"Do you think I'd let anything happen to you? This temperature just means we've got to keep you here a little longer and give you some more medicine. That's all."

A knock on the door saved me. The x-ray technician was wheeling in her machine to take a picture of Mrs. Landi's lungs as she sat propped up, and crying, in bed.

During the next four days I watched one of the curious little ironies of medicine unfold. As Mrs. Landi's white cell count climbed steadily back to normal, her pneumonia got progressively worse. The first chest x-ray, taken on Monday, had shown no unusual markings. By Friday's x-ray conference, when we put her fourth set of chest films on the board, her entire right lung field was "whited out"— obliterated by the pneumonia.

The clinical picture left no room for doubt. Her respirations were now much more frequent. Her nose flared, and she used her neck muscles to breathe. She lay quietly in bed, expending as little energy as possible. On Thursday the lab told us that the rectal swab and one blood culture had grown out pseudomonas, a particularly nasty bug if it gets in a person's lungs. By the protocol, she was already receiving the right antibiotics to attack this organism—if it indeed was the real offending party. Some virus or another bacteria could also be growing deep within the lung. All we could do was wait and watch.

As her pneumonia spread, Mrs. Landi became badly depressed. Each afternoon it became harder to cheer her up. On Tuesday we had a special talk. She began with words I would hear many times in the next two weeks.

"I never thought it would happen like this. I was never sick in my life and now this. I don't understand."

Her voice was heavy with bewilderment and resignation. She paused. Then, for the first and only time, she asked me the ultimate question.

"I'm going to die, aren't I?"

It was nearly dusk. A long, thin crimson cloud edged over West Rock. One hundred feet below her room, hospital employees were hurrying home through late January, home to the smell of steaks in passageways and the evening paper. For a few seconds I said nothing. I just stood there savoring the afternoon sky, wondering about chance. How was it that this old lady born in a village in Italy in another century had become connected in this way with me? By what karmic rule had our spirits been fused?

I felt woefully inadequate to the task, but my words seemed predestined, and they flowed easily.

"Ada, you know nobody can answer that question. You have a bad pneumonia. We are giving you our most powerful medicines. The other medicines fixed the bad blood. Now, if we can fix the lungs you will get better and go home."

"Am I going to die, soon?" she persisted.

I could no longer lie. "If your lungs don't get better, you will die."

"I never thought it would be like this. I thought it would be quick, at home." Her body lifted in a long slow shrug. "Well, you gotta take what's coming to you. That's all you can do."

She spoke in the simple words of an immigrant who had never mastered the language. Yet her voice resonated with the awful tones of the Old Testament. In grudging acquiescence, she greeted her fate. Imagine her disbelief. A month earlier she had been at work in her home. No heart attack or painful fall brought her to the hospital. She had walked in on a doctor's advice, and since that day her health had failed her.

I tried to reassure her. "Let's wait and see. Give the medicines a chance to work. We'll get you out of here."

"You'll try, Doctor Phil, I know that."

"I hope you will try too, Ada. There are lots of people who love you, who want you to get better, and to go home. Your husband, your sons."

"Yes, I love them." Then, she turned squarely to me. "I love you too," she said.

"I love you, too, Ada."

I grasped her hand tightly, and we stood there, locked in time, saying nothing. Slowly, tears welled into her eyes. With great effort she twisted her face away, seeking the privacy of her pillow, and sobbed. I stayed with her, saying nothing, until she loosened her grip. For the first and only time, I leaned over and kissed her forehead.

"Sleep well, Ada. I will see you tomorrow."

Two days later, on her twenty-sixth hospital day, Mrs. Landi went into respiratory failure. Despite the imposing array of antibiotics, pneumonia was ravaging her lungs. She was too weak to take in deep draughts of air, and there were too few healthy alveoli to take up the little oxygen that she could inhale. A critical point had been reached. Within the space of an hour Mrs. Landi changed from a woman with very bad lungs to a woman who could not breathe well enough to stay alive.

As the "blood gas" values were called in from the lab and as she deteriorated clinically, the covering intern was forced to make a crucial decision. How vigorously should he attempt to keep her alive? Although he did not know her case intimately, he knew it well enough to realize that her chances of getting better were very slim. Only two alternatives were available. He could hesitate for an hour or so. She would then suffer a respiratory arrest. Her heart and lungs would stop working. Somebody would discover her in extremis and call a "code." A horde of nurses and doctors would rush to her room. They would work feverishly to coax her back to life, but they would almost certainly fail. It would be over. Or he could play by the book. Recognizing her peril, he could transfer her to the ICU, intubate her, hook up the respirator, and hope that with rest and antibiotics her lungs would recover.

The book makes it simple. The rule states clearly: Unless the attending physician has written a DNR (do not resuscitate) order at the front of the chart every effort must be made to keep the patient alive. From the start Mrs. Landi's sons had made it very clear that despite the gravity of her illness, they wanted no effort spared in caring for their mother. Given their attitude, it was unlikely that any doctor had ever raised the extremely delicate question of a DNR order with them. She would recieve "the full court press," a bit of jargon that is particularly appropriate. Much as a losing basketball team tries desperately to get the ball in the waning seconds, the doctors would try to save her against ridiculous odds. The intern was good, and he played by the book. It only took about fifteen minutes to wheel Mrs. Landi's bed to the elevator, go up one flight to the ICU, intubate her, and hook up the respirator. In keeping with the pattern of her care, the intern did all this without consulting the patient.

The style and pace of the intensive care unit contrasted sharply with the other hospital wards. The nursing desk looked like a satellite tracking station. On a U-shaped table running the room's perimeter stood twelve cardiac monitors, one for each patient bed. Across each oscilloscope screen marched an unending signal, a medical ticker tape reporting the electrical vagaries of the heart to which it had been assigned. In the upper right-hand corner of the monitor a digital display flashed each incremental change of heart rate and blood pressure. Night never came to the ICU. Each patient needed around-the-clock care, and at any time a new "player" could arrive.

The ICU nurses were efficient and tough. Not only was their knowledge of human physiology superior to that of most floor nurses, they had developed a sixth sense for impending crisis. When a patient coded, they acted with the reflexes and alacrity of a SAC air defense team, carrying out orders before the resident had spoken. Because their patients usually stayed only a few days before being transferred to a regular bed or dying, the unit nurses seemed aloof from the drama in which they acted. For them more than for anybody else, death had become routine.

When I went in to see her for the first time it took only seconds for me to realize how dramatically Mrs. Landi's life had changed. She was in the room just opposite the nursing station. From the desk one could watch the rise and fall of the plunger that was forcing a mixture of air enriched with 40 percent oxygen through clear plastic tubing and into her lungs eight times each minute. The isolation about which I had been concerned when she had been under mask and glove precautions was insignificant compared to the isolation she must now feel. She could no longer speak. She just lay there, propped up a bit, a plastic airway in her mouth, looking at me. Never have I seen such a look of helplessness and despair. She looked like an animal caught in the steel grip of a trap and tangled in hunter's ropes. Around her bed stood three IV poles, each dangling a bag of fluid—maroon whole blood, milky white intralipid (a feeding solution, now necessary because she could no longer eat or drink), and bright yellow liquid vitamins. She was engulfed in the thin polyethylene tubing of IV lines. The steady hum of the respirator and all this medical paraphernalia made it hard to get close enough to comfort her. Despite the constant ebb and flow of nurses and doctors, Mrs. Landi was in solitary confinement.

I realized that we could no longer communicate as we had. This gentle, talkative old lady, who had been cleaning house a month ago, could now respond only with eyelids. We set up a system: One blink would mean yes, and two would mean no. But because she was very weak and hard of hearing, even this system would often fail.

One day flowed into the next, with no improvement in Mrs. Landi's clinical status and no radiological evidence that her lungs were clearing. Although we could no longer talk, I still came to her room each afternoon. I was so certain that she would soon die that I could no longer offer any real encouragement. I knew of only one way to help her. Because she could not drink any fluids, her mouth was always bone dry, so each day I brought a cup of crushed ice into her room. I would open up a piece of gauze, spoon some ice chips into it, and twist the gauze to make a mouth-sized bundle. When she saw me bring the cold wet gauze forward, she would eagerly arch open her jaws and then clamp down hard, sucking on it with the frenzy of a lost traveler who had stumbled upon an oasis in the desert. She would not relax that grip until her tongue had salvaged all the coolness that the gauze could offer. She was insatiable. Each time I pulled the gauze away and started to leave, her look beseeched me for more ice. I knew she would feel dry again in minutes, and so I felt guilty when I stopped.

I reread the last paragraph and I pause, wondering whether it is possible to tell you what those moments were really like. Alone in a hospital room I offer ice chips to a dying woman. This trivial act, taking a few minutes of my day, constitutes the one sensual pleasure left in her life, the one physical comfort in her agony. Once while doing it, I remembered that the last request made by Christ was, "I thirst." A soldier had filled a sponge with vinegar, placed it on a branch of hyssop, and offered it up to Him. After He had received the vinegar, He bowed his head and gave up His spirit. I had not thought of this story for twenty years; her suffering dug the image out of dim memories of Sunday mornings in my childhood. How laden with irony all this is, for as I compose these words I pull out my Bible, left to me by my grandmother and unopened for years, and turn briefly to the Book of John to reread this part of the crucifixion.

One of her sons was often in the room when I came to visit. Usually, he would be standing quietly at the foot of her bed, the only position where she could see him, telling her some tidbit of family news or just staring at the mysterious tubes and machines that were keeping his mother alive. As week after week had passed, they had associated me ever more closely with her care. Interns and residents frequently rotated to other hospital wards, and the sons rarely spoke to her private doctors, so they often turned to me for reports on their mother's condition. It was in talking to them that I learned the price of honesty was sometimes despair.

Their first questions were fairly easy: What did today's x-ray show? What was her platelet count? Was that a good number? Then, they got difficult. Why aren't the nurses paying more attention to her? How can she get good care if the interns keep rotating? Why aren't the antibiotics working? Finally, they became impossible. Was she ever going to get better? When would she come off the respirator? What were the odds? Was she going to die? During the first week that Mrs. Landi lay in the ICU, I held out some small measure of hope to her sons. I preferred not to deal in percentages, but I continued to say, "She has a small chance." But as her blood gases began to deteriorate and she began to require a richer and richer mixture of oxygen, I realized it was time to stop.

What was I to do? An awful cloud of secrecy had descended. Nobody involved in caring for Mrs. Landi, not the nurses, nor the house staff, nor the private doctors, held out any hope for her recovery. But the private doctors refused to confront her family. As the days passed they ordered one special consult or fancy test after another, and still they let her sons hope. The nurses were growing bitter. Seasoned by many stormy deaths, they had developed a painfully logical approach to hopeless cases. The intensive care unit housed only twelve beds, and Mrs. Landi, kept on the edge of life by a respirator, was controlling one of them. In all the other rooms patients came and went; some died and others recovered, but the drama was usually played quickly. It was against the rules of triage to lie helplessly in an expensive ICU bed week after week. On some nights all twelve beds were full; so when disaster struck, a desperately ill patient might be denied access to the special services of the unit.

It was probably not true (as a nurse urged me to believe) that salvageable lives were being lost because the doctors would not move Mrs. Landi out of the unit to die elsewhere. "They are keeping her here because they make more money that way," she argued angrily. But I was certain that this explanation made no sense. Their practice was booming, and Mrs. Landi was probably taking up an inordinate amount of their time.

As I watched the situation get steadily more tense, I became convinced that we were all trapped by the inflexibility of the system. The doctors, trained oncologists, had been taught that cancers must be treated vigorously and persistently. For them medicine was a battleground where victory, if it came at all, came after great struggle. Although they "knew" her case was hopeless, they also "knew" that sometimes they won unexpected victories. It was hard for them to quit. They could not see the case with the simple certainty of the nurses. They knew that when they gave up, they also extinguished the family's hope. In Mrs. Landi's case a decision to transfer her to a regular hospital bed would be a death sentence. The system permitted only the private physician to discuss this decision with the family. In the meantime nurses and house staff just had to wait and deal with the progressively more emotional demands of the family as best they could. It was not my place or theirs to inform the family that the kindest act would be to pursue a course of benign neglect and hope that she died quickly.

The worst day came in early March. I walked into the ICU to find that Mrs. Landi had been scheduled to undergo a bronchoscopy that morning in the operating room. Under anesthesia, a thoracic surgeon would place a long tube down her trachea and look into her lungs. He would then take a bit of tissue from several spots. The ostensible purpose was to determine if some as yet unidentified organism was merrily propagating in defiance of the many antibiotics she had received. I knew something must be afoot. I pulled aside Linda, a nurse I had befriended, and asked, "What goes?" She told me that last night one of the private doctors had finally told the sons how hopeless the situation was. He had then asked whether they wished him to transfer their mother to a private floor and write a DNR order into her chart. They had reacted very emotionally, threatening a lawsuit if she was moved out of the unit and demanding that every possible last-ditch effort be made on her behalf. The doctors had little alternative. Mrs. Landi stayed in the unit, and the bronchoscopy was scheduled on the slim chance that it would find some new diagnostic fact.

I went with her to the operating room. As he handed me the teaching scope, an instrument that allowed me to watch him maneuver inside her lungs, the surgeon was blatantly critical.

"This is one of the most pointless procedures I have ever done. This woman is at death's door, her lungs are dead, and somebody orders a bronchoscopy. How cruel!"

In his expert hands, it went quickly. The anesthesia lasted only twenty minutes, and an hour later Mrs. Landi was back in her ICU bed.

Late in the afternoon I stopped in to see her. She had been so unresponsive lately that my visits had become very mechanical. I would gently rouse her, and talk quietly of some trivial news in my life as she sucked on the gauze ice bag. Today was different. Perhaps the trauma of her trip to the operating room had squeezed one last burst of energy from her cells. She lay propped up, and her eyes followed me as I moved across the room. I had seen her face every day now for two months, and I had come to know it well. Even as it had changed, as the hair had fallen out and the cheeks had sunk, I had been able to monitor her mood by looking at her eyes. At the beginning her eyes had darted with curiosity, later they had clouded with despair; once they had lighted up with love. Today, they burned me with hatred. Although it had been weeks since she had spoken, I could hear her voice in that look.

"You promised to take care of me. You told me I would get better. Every day has gotten worse. Today was horrible. You have betrayed me."

I pretended not to notice. Carefully I spooned the ice into the gauze and offered it to her. She fixed me for a long moment with that burning stare. Then, for the first time, she turned away, refusing the ice, refusing the one succor I could offer. It was over between us. She wanted no more of me. My first impulse was to try to talk to her. But as I formed my words I suddenly realized how futile it was. We were beyond negotiation.

"I'll see you tomorrow, Ada."
I quickly left the room.

I had rehearsed the ending many times. I would walk
into the intensive care unit one afternoon and Mrs. Landi
would not be there. Some stranger would be in her bed.
The nurse would see my curious look and tell me how her
life had ended. It happened the very next day. The young
March sun shone through "her" window onto the face of
another little old lady. I paused at the door, started forward, saw the stranger, and turned to go. One of the
nurses who, I think, had watched my visits with some
sympathy came up to me. "She died at 6:30 this morning.
Her heart just started to slow down and we just watched."
"Thanks a lot," I said and walked away. It was finished.

Unlike theatrical performances, life's dramas rarely end
on cue. The stories continue and a long hiatus often
separates chapters, much as though one has put one book
aside for another. About two months after Mrs. Landi's
death I received a note from Diane, a hospital social
worker, telling me that Ray, one of her sons, wanted to
speak to me. Ray was still struggling to work through his
mother's death and to resolve some tough questions. How
did she die? Did someone decide to stop treating her?
There had occasionally been harsh words between the
family and the hospital staff. Had the interns and nurses
taken less good care of Mrs. Landi because the sons had
fought with them? Diane felt that Ray trusted me, and she
thought I could help him resolve some of the guilt that
lingered in him.
After reading the note, my first reaction was anger. I
wanted no part of this sad business. I knew that some of
Ray's questions were irrational. His mother had gotten

excellent care, and the occasional sparks between the staff
and the family were a routine part of a long, terminal stay
in a hospital. These questions I could answer. But I also
knew that the physicians involved in her care had not
painted a realistic picture of Mrs. Landi's illness for her
family. How could I now tell Ray that his mother never
really had much chance of walking out of the hospital. The
long stay had put great pressures on family finances and
divided the brothers. Ray had once accused the others,
who wanted at the end to limit the care given their mother,
of putting money ahead of her survival. He would be
hoping for answers that would justify his position. If I were
honest, I would not make him feel better. In fact, her
condition had been hopeless and a small fortune had been
squandered in the intensive care unit.

But, was it not my duty to talk to Ray? The word "doctor"
means teacher. I could help him understand. Even though
I was a lowly third-year clinical clerk, he had invested me
with the powers of a competent physician. Should I not
treat this experience as part of my own education, part of
the magical becoming that seemed to proceed in every
direction at once? And to be really truthful, did I not thirst
for the kind of power that Ray was offering me. Secretly,
did I not believe that I was more competent to help him
than any of the doctors who had been involved in the case?

We met for lunch in the hospital cafeteria. I greeted him
warmly and tried to keep the conversation light as we
moved through the crush of people in the food line. One
look at him and I knew he was depressed. The room was
crowded and I sought the end of a table where we could
have some shred of privacy. Although he had brought a
sandwich, Ray did not touch it. He pulled a crumpled
piece of paper from his pocket on which were written about
thirty questions. "You don't mind?" he asked, as I glanced
at the sheet. "There is so much I want to ask you."

We began with the details of his mother's care. A huge

abyss suddenly opened up between us. Ray asked question after question about x-rays, blood gas studies, and medicines. He had tried hard to understand his mother's care, but it was so complicated. Every observation he had made had fueled his fantasy that somewhere a therapeutic failure had occurred.

"If my Mom was having trouble getting enough oxygen, why was the dial on the machine only set at 40 percent instead of 100 percent?"

"A pure flow of oxygen over even a few days (she had been on a respirator for a month) could actually cause great harm to the lungs."

"Why did they stop taking x-rays?"

"Your mom's chest had been "whited out" for ten days when they stopped. She was on a bunch of antibiotics and she was making no progress. If she improved, we would have learned that by examining her before the x-ray pictures would change."

Next he turned to what was really bothering him. Had everyone tried their best? How come so many doctors were involved? Did people give up on her? Did the care change when the insurance money ran out? On each point I tried to reassure him, but he wasn't listening to me. Suddenly they were just spilling out; one question somersaulting after another to stand between us at the table. Then he started to talk about his brothers, and his voice broke and the tears came. By now the nurses sitting next to us were eavesdropping on our conversation. I grasped his arm and drew him to a corner of the hospital lobby.

It is not a charming place, a large high-ceilinged room dotted with vinyl furniture, but it was quiet! While he sobbed quietly, I talked about his mother's illness. Suddenly the truth seemed unimportant, all desire to criticize the way in which she was overtreated left me.

"Ray, your mother and I got to know each other well. She had good health for seventy-nine years. She had her share of sadnesses I know, but she had a good life. At the end God gave her a tough, incurable disease. It took three months for her to die, and it was horrible. But everyone, including you and your brothers, did his best. I know I can't reach your sadness, but I should be able to reach your guilt."

My little speech continued in that vein for five or ten minutes. I frankly don't know if it helped, but I gave it my all. As I talked, a third-year medical student trying to help a fifty-year-old man deal with his mother's death, my own most intimate fears danced across my brain. When and where would I sit crying while someone spoke with me about my mother? How cruel life seemed. I banished the thought and continued at my task. The hour passed, and the demands of the world intruded. I had other duties, and Ray had to get back to his job. We walked out into the hot, bright day. He took my hand.

"You are like a priest, so willing to help others."

I knew I had been given a great compliment from this good Catholic man. Suddenly, he was crying again. He choked out a good-bye and walked, head bent in sorrow, down the hill.

Chapter 8

SUBINTERNSHIP

After the challenges of the clerkship year, the fourth year of medical education is almost universally anticlimactic. Although an ample array of electives (three-week blocks of study on the renal service, in ophthalmology clinic, or reading x-rays with the radiologists) are offered, these subspecialties are so esoteric that the student is largely an observer. Typically, one might spend more time in the library reading about patients than seeing them. Unlike the clerkships, the electives carry no day-to-day responsibility for patient care. For most of us this sudden demotion from the team to consulting role was a most welcome relief.

The fourth year is one of gradual withdrawal. The student finally believes that the journey through medical school is, in fact, finite. By autumn the seniors are deeply immersed in applying to, visiting, and interviewing for residency programs. Not infrequently, this involves much time traveling, and it is not difficult to add vacation days to such trips.

The two major academic tasks in the fourth year at Yale are the preparation of a medical thesis (a requirement of few other U.S. medical schools but one common in European education) and the subinternship. The medical school thesis is not nearly as demanding as a doctoral thesis for the Ph.D. Nevertheless, the faculty expects that several months of serious effort in "original research" will yield a solid paper. There were many thesis options. One could do a retrospective "chart review" of several hundred patients in an effort to verify whether a particular set of factors influenced medical outcomes, one could do a physiology project in a basic science laboratory, one could work with the epidemiologists in the school of public health. The list was endless.

I chose a project on the history of medicine, a discipline that has departmental status at Yale. Using archival records, I spent about three months researching the history of involuntary sterilization of retarded persons in the United States—one consequence of the eugenics movement. Recalling the madness of the third year and knowing that internship was but one year away, I successfully made this period one of quiet contemplation. The rare book rooms of Yale's libraries seem to be truly in a different world from the hospitals. For me those months represented a return to life before medical school when I had spent a year as a "research fellow" completely unfettered and free to pursue studies as I wished.

It was just as I was starting my three months of thesis research, a period which for me was the first in a long time when all seemed right with the world, that I signed up (a voluntary act) to do a subinternship.

Most fourth-year students who elected to do subinternships chose internal medicine. For the people who had decided to train in surgery or obstetrics it was the last opportunity to study internal medicine. Another reason for the popularity of the medical "sub" was that the department had fostered the belief that medicine was the queen of the profession. Internal medicine was the land of the intellectual giants; here and here alone did physicians ponder pathophysiology rather than merely treat disease. Most importantly, the medicine sub offered the greatest possible opportunity for the student to act as a physician.

In its official guidelines the Department of Medicine cited four educational objectives for the subinternship:

> *First, it should provide the opportunity to increase their overall knowledge of and experience with a wide variety of disease processes. Second, the student should be able to follow more closely a larger number of patients than was possible during the clerkship. This experience should allow students to increase their clinical acumen, improve their technical skills and develop an appropriate level of clinical confidence. Third, the setting of the subinternship should develop in the student a sense of patient care responsibility beyond that experienced during medical clerkships. This increased sense of responsibility should begin with admission of the patient to the medical ward and should be maintained by the very close day-to-day interactions between the subintern and the patient. A fourth goal of medical subinternships should be to expand the opportunity for students to assess critically their own level of performance in the setting of a medical ward. This additional exposure should also give the faculty and housestaff greater opportunity to assess the students and to guide them in their future careers.*

Let there be no mistake, everyone from the Chief of Medicine to the senior residents to the "subs"—everyone, that is, except the patients—realized that the sub was not yet a physician. Indeed, the six-week rotation was intended to advance that process. The departmental guidelines tried hard to make the distinction and to protect the patient:

> *On the other hand, medical subinterns cannot be considered substitutes for first year residents. Neither attending physicians nor housestaff should expect subinterns to function at the level of first year residents, even though some students may prove capable of performing at this level. Both the number of patients assigned to subinterns and the severity of illness of assigned patients should be carefully modulated so that the student is not overwhelmed by the experience and so that patient care in no way suffers. In general, subinterns should admit and follow no more than*

one-half the number of cases assigned to a first year medical resident and under no circumstances should they admit more than 5-7 cases per week. Moreover, the formulation of a diagnosis, the ordering of laboratory tests, and the thera- peutic plan and written orders should all be discussed with the ward resident and/or attending physician before tests are ordered or orders are actually written. All written orders must be countersigned by the supervising medical resident or the attending physician before a nurse tran- scribes them. Although medical subinterns are expected to perform certain diagnostic procedures normally performed by first year residents (thoracentesis, lumbar puncture, etc.), all such procedures will be performed under the direct supervision of a physician with appropriate experi- ence.

The subinternship offers senior students the maximum possible day-to-day responsibility for the care of patients. Like interns, they see the patient first, conduct a history and physical examination, assess the patient's immediate needs, write the orders that direct the care, and plan the patient's hospital course. Students experience varying sub- internships, depending on the hospital, the specialty, and the house officers with whom they work. For example, the Department of Pediatrics offered a subinternship lasting four weeks, during which the student was on call every fourth night and did not admit patients to the ICU. Keep- ing in mind that medical students, who are assuming direct responsibility for patients for the first time, are in a mental state somewhere between fear and terror, the pediatrics sub was still considered relatively easy. Both the house staff and the nurses were very protective of the kids, the call schedule was light, and the rotation was short.

Six months later on an icy January evening just before I would start my sub, the picture was not so rosy. As I sat in my drafty apartment reading the departmental guidelines, a sinking feeling filled my stomach. Tomorrow morning I would march out of the house with my little black bag and try to pass myself off to other human beings as a doctor. I would have a better chance selling the Brooklyn Bridge. I imagined that this must be how people feel when they don a parachute and get in an airplane for their first jump.

I read the departmental guidelines over several times, but the reassuring language did not seem to offer much comfort. Remembering the great medical school aphorism that misery loves company, I decided to call Paul, who was going to work with me on this subinternship. A slight, intense guy, Paul was one of the top students. We had done a couple of third-year rotations together, and although we rarely socialized, I liked him a lot. Besides being very bright, he had a sense of humor and a certain toughness. Although we talked on the phone for only a couple of minutes, the conversation resembled the secret pacts made by Tom Sawyer and Huck Finn before they set out on a midnight adventure. Come hell or high water we were going to stick together.

I had not heard a word from anybody at the VA, so I made a point of arriving before seven-thirty. Unlike surgeons, residents in internal medicine never "rounded" before then. The hospital elevators were maddeningly slow. As I climbed the pale yellow cinder block stairway to Ward 4B, I wondered how many times I would be up and down these stairs during the next six weeks. This was my first miscalculation; I should have wondered how many ascents I would make that day!

The floor was curiously still. The nurses were "in report" (switching shifts behind closed doors), the interns had not yet arrived, and the patients were still in bed. I sauntered into the small interns' room, well known to me from other rotations. The dawn light was no match for the fluorescent glare overhead. Three small desks stood in their corners, and a half dozen cheap desk chairs of different vintages were crowded in the center of the room. A battered, unused telex machine was perched next to one desk. The only wall hangings were a chalkboard and an ancient note from the head nurse sternly ordering the interns to "clean up this room today." The room was in the usual disarray. Dirty scrub suits, paper cups, plastic syringes, photocopies of esoteric medical articles, unused needles, and a few test tubes were scattered among the candy wrappers on the desks. As it always had been in such places, my sense of order and cleanliness was instantly offended. But I knew from experience that it was pointless to clean the place up. There seemed to be an unwritten rule that the doctors' rooms had to be messy.

Ten seconds after I arrived, Paul pulled in. The conversation began on an ominous note.

"Do you know who our residents are?" asked Paul.

"No."

"Sandy Goodman and Barb Gilman. Sandy's OK. I know her. But Barb is tough as nails, real smart and a bit arrogant. She likes to put subs down."

This was worrisome news. But I remembered Barb from the prior year when she had been an intern. Although she definitely had been hard-nosed, I knew that she had liked me. I resolved to be as charming as possible, hoping that I might help my chances for survival. Only later did I realize that for the first time in my life I was using the same tactics that men often accuse women of using in the workplace. I was trying to use attractiveness as a means to succeed.

Within the next five minutes the rest of the team rolled in. Trying our best to be smooth, Paul and I greeted them in turn. The two interns with whom we would share the call schedule were Arthur Bollanyi and Clif Elwell. Art showed little interest in being friends. The first thing he did was to announce that one of the battered desks in the corner was his property. In a room where three desks were to be shared by seven people, this was an aggressive act.

Rather than argue with him, I fell into the time honored pecking order of medicine and meekly moved my belongings to another desk, mentally drawing the conclusion that he was a jerk.

It is curious how a momentary exchange like that can predict a relationship. Art, I found out, was a very smart guy. Born in Hungary, he had emigrated to the United States during his teens. He had worked hard to master English and had been a star medical student. He could have taught me a great deal, but he was too deeply enmeshed in the power politics of medicine to earn my trust. Art was the kind of guy who slaved to please those above him and abused those below him. More than once during the next six weeks he would "trash" me at rounds. Trashing is a technique by which one team member points out as subtly as possible the stupidity of another. Art was not a champion trasher because he was not nearly as subtle as he thought, but he tried.

The other intern, Clif, had graduated from Duke Medical School. He was a tall, slender guy with a great sense of humor and a superb knowledge of medicine. But, in his own words, intership had made him "toxic," a condition somewhat akin to manic-depressive illness. The periodicity of this disease varied exactly with his call schedule. I soon realized that on the morning after he had been on call, Clif had no tolerance for anyone or anything. He crawled about in a state of angry depression. During these mornings the intellectual debate that is so much a part of internal medicine made him nearly homicidal. On these days, Clif's only wish was to sip coffee in the cafeteria and fondle a pocket calendar on which he could count over and over again the number of days left in his internship. To dramatize this counting he used a spinal needle, a long, thin needle, that he carried with his pens in his breast pocket. At ID ("intern depression") rounds, held for ten minutes in the cafeteria each morning, he would unsheath his needle and obliterate the day's date from a wallet-sized calendar. Over the weeks Clif's blackly humorous tales about the horror of internship both brightened my life and clouded my future.

There were also three third-year medical students on the team. They would follow patients with the interns, so Paul and I would not work with them. Despite the fact that we moved in different orbits I paid special attention to these folks. This was my first opportunity to observe people who were behind me on the training ladder. They were a sort of reference point, reminding me how very different were the experiences of each year in medical school. They also helped to crystallize my thoughts about the medical "pecking order" and how people adapted to it.

One "stud"—as third-year clerks were called (subs were called "subhumanoids" or "slaves")—named Karen drove me crazy. She was a well-scrubbed, petite woman with sparkling blue eyes and a constant smile. She worked much harder than I ever had, and her unceasing (and successful) efforts to impress the residents made me quietly angry. The second clerk, an older guy named Lew, had adopted a different solution to the problem of being a third-year student. He projected an image of self-assurance. He was Mr. Easy, always there and never ruffled by the demands of his training. Lew was clever; he had learned the tricks early and actually worked much less than the residents thought. The third student, named Julie, was my favorite, probably because our styles were similar. She was fairly quiet at rounds, only speaking to report the progress of the patients whom she followed. She did not try to draw attention to herself, preferring to hang back. But Julie took no grief from her superiors. When they teased her, she gave as good as she got.

Rounds began that first morning at 7:45, with the seven underlings standing in a huddle around the residents. Sandy, the senior resident, had thick glasses that framed a

pretty face and an impish grin. She warmly welcomed us
and paused to make a brief effort at orientation. I liked her.
Barb was a short, dark-haired woman with a tense, hurried
manner. Her first announcement was that the subs were on
call today. My stomach fluttered. This was bad news. Not
only were Paul and I to "pick up" (take responsibility for) a
group of patients already in the "house," we would have to
admit patients that day and cover the other interns' services that night. Paul tapped me on the shoulder.

"Let's flip for the first admission."

"OK," I said. "You call it."

A nickel went spinning into the air as Paul chose,
"heads."

"Tails," I announced.

"Gee," said Paul, grinning slyly, "you get first admission."

"Paul, Paul, my boy, how could you sink so low," said I.
"I win. You go first."

Rounds lasted for two hours that morning. Starting in
the MICU and marching from bed to bed, we were introduced to thirty-five patients. Art had eighteen patients on
his service, which equaled the record at the "VA Spa." His
sole desire in life seemed to be to discharge as many of
them as quickly as possible. Besides being desolate at the
thought of being responsible for eighteen sick people, the
only other part of that morning that I remember was
meeting my first patients.

Sandy divided up the eight patients who had belonged to
the intern going off service so that Paul and I each "picked
up" four. My first patient was Jack Bodick, a pale-looking
man with watery blue eyes who sat propped up in one of
the beds in the unit. Bodick was a big-time alcoholic, a "GI
bleeder," with huge, dilated veins at the base of his esophagus, a consequence of his cirrhotic liver disease. At any
time he could bleed out from these vessels. He had
massive ascites (fluid in his abdominal cavity), which made

him look like he was about to deliver twins. He also had the gift of gab, and I liked him. Only later did I learn that he was a real sociopath, given to manipulating the people who cared for him.

My second patient was Chuck Irwin. A powerfully built black man with a shaved head and a cockeye, he reminded me vaguely of a killer in a James Bond movie. Taciturn to say the least, his silence and a contemptuous smile enhanced his macho image. He had come into the hospital because of increasing weakness and shortness of breath on exercise, a complaint suggesting that his mitral valve (the valve between the two chambers in the left side of his heart) was getting worse. He would be getting a cardiac workup. My third patient was in the next room. Bob Turci was a fifty-five-year-old merchant marine with a Clark Gable mustache, a wide smile, and a hoarse voice. An extremely heavy smoker, he had developed a cough; routine x-rays had found a mass in his left lung. A bronchoscopy had proved that he had cancer, and he was being "staged" to decide if he might be a candidate for surgery. He had a friendly, cocky way about him, and if he grasped the real meaning of his illness, he was dealing well with it. My last "pickup" was a quiet man with pneumonia who had been admitted for a ten-day treatment of intravenous antibiotics. I remember distinctly being told that he would not require too much of my time. As it turned out, Mr. Sousa took a great deal of my time and taught me a lot—about medicine and about death.

Knowing that my first admissions would demand my full attention for several hours, I started writing my "on-service" notes right after rounds. The "on-service" note is a curious document. It appears in the patient's chart right after the prior intern's "off-service" note. These notes are really intended to do the same thing: summarize for the reader the patient's illness and hospital course up to that day. Why have two such similar notes back to back? The standard answer is that the chart is a legal document, whereas the signed note "proves" that the intern is doing his or her job. The "on-service" note is also part of the practice of "buffing" the chart. It looks good, even though it is often merely a restatement of the prior note, written before the newcomer has had much contact with the patient. About a week into my subinternship I reread my four on-service notes. The first had run about three pages. It was neatly written, followed a chronological order, and accurately summarized the patient's condition. The second, written at six o'clock in the evening, ran a page and a half. It was legible and accurate. The fourth, written about four in the morning, was a couple of paragraphs. It was a poor abstract of the preceding note, written without reviewing patient or chart.

I got my first admission at eight o'clock that evening. Sandy, the "admitting" resident, summed him up in a few seconds.

"His name is Robert Stephens. He is a sixty-four-year-old black man with cancer of the prostate that has spread everywhere. He had right-sided chest pain and cough. He has either got a pneumonia or a PE [pulmonary embolus—a clot blocking of pulmonary vessels]. He is already on the floor. Call me when you are ready to write orders."

She handed me a little white card with his ID number stamped on it and hurried off to the next admission. This was it. I grabbed my instruments and hurried off to meet him.

I found Mr. Stephens hunched over in bed, sweating profusely, and taking about forty breaths a minute. I knew in an instant that this man was definitely too sick for me. I wanted to run, but had no exit. I had to go forward. Following rules I had been taught, I politely introduced myself and tried to take a history. As a second-year student

I had been trained to take extremely thorough histories. The process had often taken an hour, leaving no part of the patient's past uninvestigated. But here was a patient who could barely talk and who needed treatment now. The history taking lasted about five minutes. I learned that he lived in the T building (a chronic care facility on the hospital grounds), that he was in chronic pain from his cancer, and that he had had a new chest pain, cough, and a temperature for two days.

I had never examined someone like him before. No matter how gingerly I moved him about, I hurt him. (Later, his x-rays showed why: His bones were simply riddled with cancer.) Every time that *he* cried out the situation became steadily more stressful for *me!* I decided to curtail my exam, focusing just on the heart, lungs, abdomen, and legs. I wanted to get the workup done so I could get the orders written. The residents had decided the therapeutic plan for this man in the emergency room: He would be "fully cultured," covered (with antibiotics) for pneumonia, and started on anticoagulant therapy because of the risk of emboli. What was I doing, beside causing him pain?

The fever workup was my job. I could at least do that; it meant getting a sterile urine sample, blood cultures, a conjunctival culture (he had pus running out of a lower eyelid), and a sputum sample. There were also the standard "admission" tests for which I had to draw some blood. Gently, I rolled up his pajama sleeve and began looking for veins. He had plump arms and dark skin, and there was not a vein in sight. After searching both arms I found one small vessel that I thought I could hit. Armed with a "butterfly," a tiny needle hooked to tubing that attaches to a syringe, I tried three times and failed.

At that point, feeling totally incompetent, I went with my tail between my legs looking for Sandy. She was at the nursing station writing an admission note. One look at me must have told her a lot. Before I could say a word, she spoke.

"This is going to be the second worst night of your life. You are going to do everything wrong. Your worst night will come next July when you are an intern. Now, tell me, what's the matter?"

"Everything. I can't even draw his blood."

"OK. Let's go do it together."

For the rest of that night Sandy was great. An hour later when I failed to place the IV line that Mr. Stephens needed for his heparin (anticoagulant) therapy, Sandy came down and put it in on her first try. Seeing no vein anywhere, I judged this just short of miraculous. Next she sat down with me and went over my orders, reminded me about what I had omitted, discussed the use of bronchodilator therapy in a patient who was wheezing, and taught me how to manage a heparin drip. I could not thank her enough.

The panic and despair I felt at having flubbed my first admission was only the beginning. When Art "signed out" to me at seven o'clock he had handed me a paper on which were scrawled the names, diagnoses, and most likely "acute" problems that might befall the patients for whom he was responsible. Until rounds the next morning I could be called for any matter—from a trivial complaint like difficulty falling asleep to a life-threatening crisis. Having never "covered" before, I did not know what to expect.

It was around nine o'clock, as I was trying to write some orders for Mr. Stephens, that I first heard my name blare over the overhead page system. "Dr. Reilly, please call 769. Dr. Philip Reilly, please call 769." A frisson of terror scampered up my back. Extension 769 was the phone in the intensive care unit. What horrible task did the unit nurses want me to perform? I grabbed the nearest phone and dutifully answered.

"This is Phil Reilly." I could not bring myself to say Dr. Reilly, I most certainly did not feel like a physician.

"Dr. Reilly, Mr. Ruggiero is having quite a bit of ectopy, and his tracing does not look right. Would you please take a look at his Swan?"

My worst fears had been realized. A Swan-Ganz catheter is a long, hollow tube that may be used to measure filling pressures in the pulmonary vessels. It is inserted into a large vein and threaded into the right side of the heart and through the valves, until its tip lies in the pulmonary artery. Sometimes the tip of the catheter floats into undesirable or dangerous positions. If it lodges against the inside of the right ventricular wall, it can irritate the muscle and cause irregular beats (ectopy). Although this is not immediately dangerous, it increases the risk of a patient going into a life-threatening heart rhythm. It definitely requires attention—in this case by me.

Trying to look as intelligent and relaxed as possible, a subterfuge that could not possibly fool the unit nurses, who had seen scores of subs come and go and who most certainly knew that I was terrified, I went to Mr. Ruggiero's bedside. The monitor above his bed was faithfully recording a PVC (premature ventricular contraction) about every six seconds. As the nurse had said, the pressure tracing did not have the expected wave form. With the nurse, a twenty-year veteran standing next to me, I gazed dumbly at the oscilloscope, wondering just what was the proper way to pull back a Swan. I suddenly realized that I was not even sure which of the several lines running into his arm (which was wrapped in gauze and tape and strapped to a board) was in fact the Swan. I decided to retreat. Afraid to admit my complete ignorance, I lied.

"Yes, this needs repositioning. I'll be back in about five minutes, as soon as I finish with another patient."

There was no other patient. As soon as I fled from the ICU I went to a phone and beeped the resident. I needed some quick guidance. To my surprise, the chief resident, who had lectured to me a year ago about the uses of the

Swan-Ganz catheter, answered the page. Asking him what to do seemed like an admission of complete stupidity. Only by reminding myself that the patient had an unquestionable right not to have a buffoon tugging on a tube inside his heart was I able to proceed. He listened politely to my recapitulation of the problem. He then said, in his laconic way, "I guess you better pull it back a couple of inches." Before I could say anything else there was a click followed by a very loud silence.

There was no choice but to get on with it. I still had to perform gram stains on Mr. Stephen's various bodily fluids (a critically important task, as it would guide the initial choice of antibiotics), and at any time another patient could arrive. Time was precious. Armed with a scissors I slinked stealthily past the unit nursing station. Mr. Ruggiero was asleep. He reminded me of the giant captured by the Lilliputians. Hoping not to dislodge the skein of lines in which he was tangled, I began cutting away gauze and tape from his arm. I found the Swan's pressure transducer attached to the catheter in the crook of his right arm. The rest had to be performed under sterile conditions. After donning gloves and with one eye cocked watchfully on the monitor, I grasped the catheter and began to pull ever so gently. I uttered a silent prayer that I would not start some horrible ventricular rhythm. A half inch, an inch, two inches. Miraculously, nothing had happened, except that two huge drops of sweat were trickling down my glasses. As I retaped the catheter in place, I felt a presence. One of the nurses was grinning at me from the doorway.

"Good job," she said. "I'll finish taping. Don't forget to order an x-ray."

Of course, I had not thought of that. The chest x-ray would tell us where the catheter tip now sat. Later that night when I finally read the x-ray I saw that the tip did appear to be in the right ventricle. I made a mental note that never again would I have to reposition a Swan for the first time.

The hours between ten o'clock and two o'clock flew. My life became an endless series of short errands. Mr. Verdi needed a sleeping pill. Mr. Savin had a belly-ache. Mr. Fleishman had a temperature of 101.6. Each of these problems required evaluation and a decision. I knew that even something as simple as a decision to order a sleeping medication could trigger an iatrogenic disaster. A belly-ache could be a demand for attention by a scared patient or a hint of impending catastrophe such as ischemic colitis. A fever workup meant an hour of "scut." I had to collect all the relevant bodily fluids (blood, urine, sputum), gram stain them, culture them, and decide whether to initiate other therapy. The patients were on the fifth floor and the labs, on the first floor. As the night wore on the stairs acquired mythic significance. I was Sisyphus, and this was my purgatory.

By two in the morning my toes were blistered, my calves were aching, my hands were stained in wild patterns of red and purple by Gram's reagents. I reeked of body odor and wanted more than anything else in the world to go home and sleep. As I sat at a desk clutching a styrofoam cup filled with tepid vending machine coffee, I tried to confront the awful fact that I had voluntarily entered into an agreement, the terms of which forbade me to leave the hospital for at least another sixteen hours. This was unquestionably the most masochistic act I had ever committed. Fantasies of rebellion began to stir in my soul. Deep inside a voice whispered, "You can leave right now. No one can make you stay. Why, it would not even prevent you from graduating. You don't have to do this. Go home." Everything the voice had whispered was true.

It was fitting that this fantasy was interrupted by a call from the ER. My next admission had arrived. Suddenly my tune shifted. There was clearly no escape. I glanced at my watch—2:16 in the morning. I had five hours in which to work up and write up this new patient. It would take me at least three hours to get everything done. All hope for sleep vanished.

The rest of my first night was punctuated by sleep-deprived hallucinations. I felt more like a sleep-starved trucker making a transcontinental run than a young doctor. I was too exhausted to be worried about my competence or what the nurses or anybody else thought of me. My new patient was Mr. Grupp, an ancient, emaciated, nearly comatose man who had been shipped in from a nursing home with a fever. He had pneumonia, and his labored breathing told me he could decompensate and die at any time. That was fine with me. At three o'clock in the morning as I stood over his bedside starting an IV he was an enemy, part of the plot to deprive me of sleep. If he died, I could sleep for an hour. If he lived, I would be up all night. He lived, and I spent the hour from five to six pouring over his thick records (he had been admitted with pneumonia three times in the last eight months) and writing my note.

Morning (my second morning there) brought no relief. Oblivious to my personal hell, the team assembled, rounded, and dispersed to regular chores. It was under-stood that Paul and I would work for yet another ten hours before crawling home to bed. I stumbled through the day obsessively pondering a single question. How could a human being possibly do this for an entire year of intern-ship?

Looking back at my six weeks as a subintern reminds me of early childhood when, newly mobile and equipped with language, the toddler begins rapidly to expand the fron-tiers of his known world. Literally everything demands to be seen, touched, smelled, tasted, and tested for the first time. The subintern's world is substantially less sensual than the child's, but there is a strange congruency in its novelty. I never knew what might happen next. Each patient entered onto my service with a set of problems that I had to confront directly for the first time. Each phone call announced a new crisis. I began to hunger for the experience that would make things routine.

Despite the daily revelations of my ignorance, I learned an immense amount in a few weeks. There were three kinds of knowledge with which I had most often to contend: facts ascertainable by history and physical examination, the diagnostic and therapeutic choices that should be made on the basis of those, and observations about the way people (patients, families, and doctors) face suffering and death. Reflections on medical education tend to focus on the process of mastering technical skills, but I believe that it was my involvement with the "management" of suffering and death during my sub that had the greatest impact on my training as a physician.

I have never been to a funeral. Once in high school I attended a wake. An older brother of a classmate had died, and motivated by some vague sense of duty and an anxious curiosity, I paid my respects to the family of a young man I barely knew. Before starting medical school I had never witnessed a death. During the second year course in pathology I attended a number of autopsies. But a corpse has a neutral quality, and in the morgue death seems, despite its propinquity, distant. During my third-year clerkships I gradually grew familiar with dying, but (with the exception of my time with Mrs. Landi) I still knew it largely at a distance. After all, I had no direct responsibility for the care of those who died.

During my six-week tour of duty as a subintern at the West Haven VA Hospital I admitted eighteen patients. Four died. Of the eighteen patients that Paul, my fellow

sub, admitted, two died. In that brief sojourn into clinical
medicine I probably witnessed a dozen deaths. I do not
completely understand the ways in which these experiences have changed my view of the world. But I am
convinced that the period in a student-doctor's training
when dying finally becomes palpable constitutes the most
significant aspect of his or her metamorphosis.

Physicians must become familiar with dying—its look,
its odor, and its sound. They must get used to the special
and onerous duties that death generates: holding the hand
of a dying patient, making the phone call to give the news
(sometimes long awaited, sometimes crushingly sudden) of
a person's death to relatives, filling out death certificates.
Physicians must contain and control their emotions and
recognize that these changes set them apart. They must
admit they are no longer uncomfortable with death, that in
many cases death seems to be the preferred outcome for a
patient, that sometimes (consciously or unconsciously) they
act or fail to act in order to increase the chance that death
will win its struggle with the patient, that they may be too
tired or busy or angry to care if a patient dies. Physicians
also must learn that other people (doctors, nurses, patients, kin) have different ways of dealing with death. Each
time that death enters the scene, to acknowledge its presence, a physician may have to remember how it felt when
it was still a new experience. Several patients taught me
about death; let me share the learning with you.

Mr. Levin was the first patient on my service who died.
He was an eighty-four-year-old man from a nursing home
who had developed a big pneumonia. As with most patients his age, Mr. Levin had a long list of medical problems. I remember thinking as I read over his chart that his
left-sided paralysis, heart disease, emphysema, and anemia
made him an unlikely prospect for much functional improvement. Regardless of how well he did in the hospital,
he would merely return to lie quietly in his nursing home

bed. We started Mr. Levin on antibiotics and hydration. He held his own for the first day, but his heavily labored breathing did not improve.

Although no family members had been contacted to discuss the question, I could tell at rounds on the morning after his admission that no one wanted to push too hard with Mr. Levin's treatment. Everyone agreed that he was the classic "gome," who would die of pneumonia either now or next time or the time after that. Tom, one of the new residents who had come on service at the end of my second week, admonished me, "Don't push too hard, Phil."

Rounds ended and I went to draw Mr. Levin's blood so I could recheck his white count (an index of infection). When I barged in, I surprised an elderly man standing, cap in hand, at the foot of the bed. One glance told me a lot. The physical similarity overrode the effects of time. This was my patient's brother. He wanted to talk, but there was no need to step out of the room. His brother, barely responsive to pain, focused every ounce of his strength on drawing in enough air to stay alive. Sometimes a few words can cover a lot of ground. I answered the man's questions as best I could.

"How bad is he?"

"Your brother had a bad pneumonia. He is very weak. We are giving him two different antibiotics by vein. They are the best we have. The big question is whether he should be put on a respirator if he fails to get enough oxygen to his tissues with just this face mask."

I had spoken slowly and deliberately, trying to convey the gravity of the situation. Now I paused, letting the message sink deep into his cortex.

"What do you think, Mr. Levin?"

"Well, Doc, he has so many other problems, and he just lies in bed in that nursing home. I don't think the oxygen machine will do anything but prolong his agony."

"I think you are right, sir. We will stick by your wishes.

Now, if you will just wait outside for a few minutes, I'll draw some blood and then you can come back in."

The whole conversation had lasted no more than a couple of minutes.

After Mr. Levin stepped outside I turned to the business at hand. He was an emaciated old guy with veins like wire cords that kept rolling from my needle. I bent over his arm, coaxing the veins. The only sound in the room was his rapid, labored breathing. He had been going at about 30 a minute since being admitted. Suddenly, while I was drawing the blood, the room changed. It took me a few seconds to realize what had happened. His breathing rate was diminishing rapidly. The breaths became slower and deeper. In less than a minute his rate dropped to 6. His breaths were now noisy gasps. He was agonal. There were several long slow breaths, then he stopped. I felt his pulse. Nothing. I put my stethoscope to his chest. No sound. I pinched his skin very hard. No withdrawal. Mr. Levin was dead. It was as though he had overheard me talking to his brother and had decided to cast his vote against the respirator.

My next two thoughts are still crystal clear. Should I call a code? Despite the fact that I was his only chance for resuscitation in the waning minutes before his brain cells would shut down irreversibly, I stood firm. A code was pointless. At best it would lead to a respirator from which he would never be weaned. Besides, his brother had just told me that he did not want to go that route. My second thought told me a lot about myself: What if he is not really dead? This, I admit, was an absurd thought. But nothing could better illustrate the level of my clinical uncertainty or my inability to accept death. Despite the obvious clinical signs, I felt an overwhelming need for corroboration. I hurried out of the room to find a doctor! Fortunately, Mr. Levin's brother was at the other end of the hall and an intern who I knew was in the next doorway. I felt like a complete idiot.

"Vinny," I asked, "I know this sounds crazy, but will you just look at this guy and make sure he's dead. He's a "no code" and he stopped breathing while I was drawing his blood."

"Sure," said Vinny, suppressing most of a gentle grin. Vinny did what I had done and agreed with my impression. Mr. Levin was dead.

The next task was to tell his brother. Ten minutes earlier he had been standing at the bedside. I had evicted him from the room, and now the man he had come to visit, his brother of eight decades, perhaps the person he loved most in the world, was dead. How would he react?

I found him glancing out of a window at the end of the corridor.

"Sir, your brother just died a moment ago. It was quite simple. He just stopped breathing."

The silence was embarrassing. Mr. Levin did not know what to do.

"Would you like to see him again?"

As though given an order, he started down the hall to his dead brother's room. He was as bewildered by death as was I. Here was a social situation for which we had no manners, no safe, programmed set of signals. Feeling an odd sense of embarrassment, I stepped out of the room. The visit lasted only a minute or two. He shuffled out looking confused, bid me good-bye, and started down the hall. He had gone but a few steps when he stopped and turned.

"What do I do about the body?" he asked.

It dawned on me that I had not the slightest idea. But I finessed an answer. "You'll have to call a funeral home. The clerk at the nursing station will give you all the details."

My momentary inability to accept Mr. Levin's death, a death that occurred in my very arms, before my very eyes, and that was witnessed by my own instruments, showed dramatically the power of the mind to deny what it does not wish to believe. It also proved to me that although the process of dying may be lengthy, death is but an instant in time.

Mr. Garabedian taught me a different lesson. Although he was not my patient, I got to know Mr. Garabedian well. His story was so tragic that no one who met him could ignore it. To this day he reminds me of the story of Job. As a young man he had been a successful political reporter for a city newspaper. He had liked his work and done it well, rising steadily in the ranks not by strategy or subterfuge, but because he worked hard. When he was forty, doctors discovered that he had glaucoma. The disease was relentless, and two years later he was blind. By forty-four he was afflicted with severe arthritis, and that disease also progressed in an unusually malignant fashion. Now at the age of fifty-four, Mr. Garabedian's joints were twisted beyond recognition. Weighing only eighty pounds, he lay in bed like a broken doll. Huge ulcerated bed sores had eroded his knees and elbows. He looked like a man who had been smote with boils.

One night as I was walking past his room, he called out for help. I went to his side. He lay in bed, listening to the scratchy music from an inexpensive transistor radio, his sole diversion through many sleepless hours.

"How can I help you, sir?"

"Could I have a sip of Seven-Up, please."

He had no use of his hands so I held the can for him while he sipped hungrily at the straw. His polite manners intrigued me, for if ever there was a patient who I expected to be angry and demanding, it was he. After that night I visited him each night that I was on call in the hospital. At the very least I made sure that he got to sip the soft drinks he enjoyed so much.

One night I could resist no longer. I railed against his misfortune. It all seemed so unfair. His answer was brief.

"I had a pretty good life until I was forty," said he. "But it's over now, and there is nothing left for me but waiting. I can't change anything. I have no power at all."

I wondered if this meant that Mr. Garabedian had asked to be given "no code" status. When I reviewed his chart, I found no formal statement on that subject. Officially, if he needed it, he was to get full resuscitative efforts.

During the next few days I began to realize how uncomfortable the ward team and nurses were with him. Unlike our visits to the other patients, no more than two of us ever visited Mr. Garabedian's room at rounds. People seemed unwilling to admit that such horrors had been heaped on him. One day at rounds I asked about his code status. Art, the intern responsible for his care, said that he had talked it over with the family and that they did not want him to be intubated. This was odd. Mr. Garabedian was an intelligent man. Why had not Art talked directly with him? I did not ask, but I suspected that Art felt too uncomfortable to discuss death so openly with a patient. Unlike the majority of patients about whom he considered code decisions, this man was well oriented and alert. The more I thought about it the angrier I became that no one had respected his dignity enough to ask Mr. Garabedian what he wished us to do.

Beside his other problems Mr. Garabedian had congestive heart failure. He frequently went into pulmonary edema (a life-threatening emergency in which fluid fills the lungs due to the weakened heart's inability to pump blood through the body), but in the past he had responded well to medical therapy. We knew that if we did not treat an episode of pulmonary edema, his long wait for death would end.

It happened at rounds one morning. as we worked our way down the corridor toward his room, we could hear him gasping for air. Sandy, the senior resident, ordered us to stay put, broke from the group, jogged to his door, and peeked in at him. After a minute or two in Mr. Garabedian's room she closed the door all but a crack and returned to the group. There was a slightly conspiratorial tone to her voice.

"He doesn't want to fight anymore," she said. "The only medicine that he wants is a little morphine so he won't be in agony, and he's going to die." She scurried off to the nursing station.

One-half hour later, as our group edged toward his room, something happened that shocked me. First one intern and then several medical students cracked jokes about Mr. Garabedian's death. They were "in" jokes from which only house officers can dissect the humor.

"Let's write transfer orders to the ECU [eternal care unit]," punned someone.

People were actually giggling about a man's impending death while he lay twenty feet away gasping for air. I was disgusted and furious. I could feel my voice quiver.

"Do you really think this is funny," I challenged.

"Calm down, Phil," said Sandy. "No one ever handles these things properly."

"Christ, Sandy, he can hear us."

"I don't think so. He's agonal."

Mr. Garabedian died a minute or so after my bitter exchange with the team. His dying and death made palpable for me the aphorism that there are circumstances under which it is wrong for a physician to prolong a person's life. The newspapers routinely carry articles about "living wills," essays about euthanasia and stories of mercy killings. But a vast moral and emotional chasm yawns between armchair reading and the duty to make decisions. The ethical rule of thumb is that if you do not know a patient's wishes, act to resuscitate him. Yet, I could not in good conscience have resuscitated Mr. Garabedian unless he had at some earlier time unequivocally ordered me to do so. Further, the way in which our team, composed of nine bright, highly educated, caring persons, handled Mr. Garabedian's death also convinced me that something very important was missing from medical training. House officers sometimes do not show enough respect for their patients. Two years of 100-hour workweeks and significant sleep deprivation make new physicians technically proficient, but the demands that hone their diagnostic and therapeutic skills leave little time to nurture their compassion.

The most troublesome experience of my subinternship was a code that was called at three o'clock one morning. At the time I was in the intern's on-call room, located at the far end of one of the ward corridors. In keeping with the rest of the subinternship, the room was devoid of all amenities. The windows were stuck shut and the thermostat was jammed permanently at 80. The mattress on the ancient bed was wrapped in a thick coat of plastic that made strange high-pitched noises each time I rolled over. Despite these discomforts, I had fallen asleep soon after hittng the pillow at about two o'clock. I was in deep REM sleep when the dreaded audio screamed the alarm: "Code 5.G4 East. Code 5.G4 East. Code 5.G4 East." As the loudspeaker wrenched me out of sleep, I noticed first that I was sweating heavily. By the time my feet hit the floor, my pulse was pounding. Muttering an endless series of obscenities, I raced down the corridor to the stairway. The code was one flight above on the surgical ward.

A code conducted at three A.M. is very different from a daytime crisis. You do not know until you get to the room whether there will be enough people to manage the problem. I arrived maybe two minutes after the code was called to find a team of six (doctors, nurses, and a respiratory therapist) huddled around an old man. Paul, the other sub, was pumping his chest. A single glance told me this was an absurd code. The "patient" had the odd grey-blue color of an old man who has been dead for a while. Paul's glance to me confirmed my opinion.

I stood at the end of the bed taking in the scene. The respiratory therapist was bag breathing the man, a third-year medical student was trying to do a femoral "stick" (to get arterial blood in order to measure its oxygen content). An IV had been started, and the medical resident was "pushing" the standard prepackaged ampules of sodium bicarbonate and epinephrine. The surgical resident was placing a central line in the man's subclavian vein. A nurse was watching the paper curl off the EKG machine waiting for signs of a ventricular rhythm. But the line was flat. I asked a floor nurse what had happened. She said that on a routine room check she had found this eighty-nine-year-old man without a respiratory rate or a pulse and had called the code. I held my tongue. We were working on a dead man. I wondered how long this would continue.

Paul was getting tired. Against my better judgment I took over the task of compressing the dead man's chest about once a second. When CPR (cardiopulmonary resuscitation) is taught, much is made of the importance of the rescuer's position. He should be perched high over the chest wall with ample room to lock his elbows and use his body weight to deliver the chest compression. I was perched precariously on the edge of the bed, buffeted by other people as they frantically tried to give various medications and place new lines. I could barely lock my arms. Nevertheless I pumped for one minute, five minutes, ten minutes. My arms were aching. Paul was gone. (Did he sneak back to bed? I wondered.) There was no one there to help me. Instead the respiratory therapist and the surgical resident offered a desultory critique of my technique. According to them, I was guilty of applying "too much torque." My arms were rotating slightly as I compressed the chest wall; this diminished the force vector intended to squeeze the blood out of the heart. "Those jerks," I thought. But I was too tired to argue.

After about fifteen minutes the scene drifted into absurdity. The surgical resident and the medical resident started to argue about the code. By now everyone agreed the man was dead, but the surgeon, who was technically in charge (the patient was under his care), would not order us to stop until he had heard from his chief resident, whom he had asked a nurse to call at home. This was because the chief resident had operated a few days earlier on the patient. While they argued, I watched a third-year student, who had no idea about what he was doing, try to place a transthoracic pacing wire. The procedure consists of inserting a long cardiac needle below the xiphoid (the tip of the breast bone) and advancing it into the heart wall. Except for me, no one was watching as the student jammed the big cardiac needle into the patient's chest. The respira-·tory therapist and I kept going through the motions of CPR, but no one was looking at the EKG recording. Finally, I could not stand it anymore. I had been pumping the chest of a dead man for twenty-five minutes. Without saying a word, I stopped, backed off the bed and stalked out of the room. No one took my place. The code was over.

Once just before I started my third year of medical school my father, a general surgeon, offered some advice.

"When someone is ready to die," he said, "there is not a doctor on earth who can stop him. Remember that, and don't ever feel guilty when you lose a patient for whom you did your best."

Mr. Sousa was the patient who proved to me the wisdom

of this advice. When Barb assigned him to my "service" the first morning of my sub, she said reassuringly, "Mr. Sousa's on two weeks of IV antibiotics for pneumococcal pneumonia. He's on auto pilot, so there's not much for you to worry about."

When I went back to talk to Mr. Sousa, it certainly appeared that Barb's assessment was correct. He was sitting in a chair, reading a novel. With his wire-rim glasses perched precariously at the tip of his nose, he looked like a college professor enjoying a quiet Sunday while the family was at church.

Because he had already been in the hospital for a week, and was scheduled to leave a week later, I did not perform an extensive history or physical. Except for the fact that he had been started on digitalis (a heart medicine used to increase the efficiency of the pumping action) a few weeks earlier, he denied having any serious medical problems. He did tell me that he had experienced periods of deep depression and had (years earlier) once been hospitalized for several months after attempting suicide. He had also taken antidepressant medicines for several years, but not recently. After spending an hour talking to Mr. Sousa and examining him, I was able to make only one significant observation. Although he used the words of an intelligent man, they rang out with a curiously flat tone.

"Everything is fine," he said, flashing a toothy, forced smile. "No, nothing you can help me with, Doc."

Two days later things began to go wrong. As I was doing my daily physical exam of Mr. Sousa I noticed that the left side of his back was "dull to percussion" (my tapping fingers did not elicit the resonant, drumlike sound expected from a normal lung field). A chest x-ray confirmed that he had developed a pleural effusion (a collection of liquid around the outside of the lung). This was not uncommon in cases of pneumococcal pneumonia, but it had happened rather late in the course of his treatment. I told Barb, and after reviewing the chest x-ray together, we decided to drain some of the fluid from the space around his lung.

This procedure, known as a thoracentesis, involves putting a needle between the ribs into the fluid-filled space, taking care not to puncture the delicate lung tissue. Yale students admit to knowing only a few critical bits of anatomical knowledge, but one is that the needle should always be inserted just above the rib because the intercostal blood vessels run along its lower margin. We performed the "tap" without incident, drawing off a quart of straw-colored liquid. I sent off some of it for lab studies that might tell us whether an infection was brewing there and flushed the rest down a toilet. Mr. Sousa had not had much trouble undergoing the procedure, and he still did not seem very sick.

When I visited him the next day, I found Mr. Sousa vomiting and doubled over in pain. He told me he had vomited five times that afternoon, but had not called for a nurse. My spirits sank. His gastrointestinal illness would have to be worked up, so any hope of going home at a reasonable hour vanished. After talking the case over with the resident, I stopped the medication order for digitalis, forbid Mr. Sousa to take in any food or liquid, "put down" a nasogastric tube (an unpleasant job in which the tube is threaded through the nose and down the esophagus while the patient helps it along by swallowing sips of water), called for a surgical consult, and sent Mr. Sousa to radiology for an "upper GI series." If you vomit at home, you have the flu; if you vomit in the hospital, you have a small bowel obstruction. The index of suspicion is dramatically different. All the studies and examinations were normal when I finally left the hospital at nine o'clock. Mr. Sousa had not vomited for five hours. He was sitting in bed reading; the only sign of change was the tube running out his nose to a suction pump on the wall.

Two days later when I again went to examine Mr. Sousa I

found yet another development. His pulse was now irregular. I found an EKG machine and took a reading. He was in atrial fibrillation (a condition in which the atria, the small upper chambers that direct blood into the muscular ventricles, are beating fast and erratically). When he had not converted to a normal rhythm by the next morning, the resident decided that he should be cardioverted.

Cardioversion sounds simple enough. A relatively weak electrical shock applied momentarily to the chest wall will depolarize the cells in the heart that "pace" its rhythm. During repolarization the normal pacing cells usually take over from the cells that have been causing the fibrillation. Because there is a small risk of a big disaster associated with cardioversion, it is undertaken with lots of precautions. To cardiovert Mr. Sousa, we moved him to the coronary care unit. The nurses placed him on a bed with a wooden board overlying the mattress and hooked him up to a cardiac monitor. An anesthesiologist then "snowed" him with a short-acting but powerful anesthetic. There were about eight people in the little coronary care unit bedroom. I found the hum of activity disconcerting and opted to hang back and watch, rather than get too involved. After all, what did I know? What help could I be? Everything was ready. Just then Allen Bair, the attending cardiologist, spied me in the corner. "OK, Phil," he said, "why don't you cardiovert your patient." My pulse rate doubled.

The defibrillator looks like something that a "stereo" nut would buy as an accessory for his system. It is about the size of a standard amplifier and has a console laden with knobs and switches. The only difference is that from each side run two curled cords (like on your telephone), each connecting to a paddle. The paddles are the size and shape of a hair brush and on the back of each is a little red button. To cardiovert a patient the operator places one paddle over the surface of the heart and the other at right angles to it (just below the armpit). After making sure that nobody (including himself) is in danger of getting shocked, the doctor presses the paddles firmly against the skin and hits the buttons.

The procedure lasted only a few seconds but it seemed much longer. Everyone in the room seemed to be giving me advice.

"Check the setting."

"Make sure nobody is touching the bed."

"Hold the paddles firmly."

"OK. Zap him."

I did. Mr. Sousa's body went rigid; his back seemed to arch as though he were levitating off the bed. Then a second later he relaxed. I looked at the monitor. He had converted to a normal sinus rhythm. I looked dumbly down at the paddles in my hands.

"Would anyone care to cardiovert the medical student?" I asked.

After Mr. Sousa had gone into atrial fibrillation, I took a much closer look at his old medical records. I realized that his heart disease was much worse than I had suspected. He had cardiomyopathy. As we talked, I realized that he must be hiding parts of his medical history from me. I decided to call his ex-wife. She told me that he had put away a fifth of whiskey daily for the last ten years of their marriage. Alcohol is a major cause of cardiomyopathy. Gradually, my unpracticed clinical eye began to see that this was no simple case of pneumococcal pneumonia. This was a case of pneumonia in a man with marginal cardiac reserve. He could tip over the edge at any time.

Two days later he fell off the edge. I was called to see Mr. Sousa at two P.M. His blood pressure and heart rate had both been declining during the day (a somewhat paradoxical situation, the heart rate usually increases). He lay in bed, in no apparent discomfort, complaining only of being hungry and feeling weak. When his blood pressure fell to 80 we moved him to the CCU. He seemed completely amenable to this change, asked few questions, and continued his long hours of reading.

He took a major turn for the worse at four A.M. the next morning. His pressure, now very low, started to fall again. Five minutes after the nurses called me to the CCU, I knew that I was in over my head. Mr. Sousa was fixing to die. I paged the resident. The next two hours were a madhouse. While Mr. Sousa lay calmly in bed, the resident, perplexed by the clinical situation, made the decisions while I did the scut work (blood culture, blood tests, blood gases). We covered him with three antibiotics, gave him steroids, and pushed fluids and pressors (drugs that constrict the arteries) to elevate his blood pressure. At six A.M. Mr. Sousa asked me to take off his wrist watch and tape it to the wall where he could see it. His speech was becoming slurred, and his mental status was changing.

"How much time do I have?" he asked. "Three weeks?"

By this time it was obvious that he was not going to survive. Nevertheless, I told the proper lie.

"I don't know. Let's make it longer than that."

The curious thing about the last day of his life was that Mr. Sousa remained quite indifferent to his impending death. He seemed totally accepting, as though he had no will to live. When I came into work the next morning he was gone. Both the CCU nurse and the intern described his death in the most bizarre way. They said his death had been "beautiful." Beginning at about three A.M. his cardiac rhythm had begun to change. Over the next twenty minutes his heart performed what Clif described as an electrical "ballet." It danced every step in its physiological repertoire, all of which had been neatly displayed on the oscilloscope. The intern and nurse had watched the monitor with fascination while Mr. Sousa, already on a respirator and receiving maximum medical therapy, had died.

Mr. Sousa taught me never to underestimate an illness. This is probably the single most important lesson that doctors need to learn. Of course, it has extraordinary implications. It means that physicians must live in a constant state of uncertainty; they can never completely forget the patients for whom they are caring. In the midst of the most relaxed moment a nagging doubt may surface; they will worry like a dog with a bone until they can thoroughly check the question. Frankly, it is a lesson that at times I resent having had to learn. It seems unfair that a physician should always have to be that preoccupied. Mr. Sousa also made me wonder if the patient's "will" to live just might matter as much as some of the folks in "holistic" medicine argue. He had arrived with a treatable illness and declined steadily regardless of our best medical efforts. He just was not interested in living.

If there is a single experience that sets physicians apart, that isolates them in a unique and lofty loneliness, it is the task of acknowledging to a patient that he or she is going to die. This duty is always sad, but when the patient perceives the complaint as relatively benign and requiring attention mainly because it persists, the duty of pronouncing a death sentence is especially odious. The news is so profoundly unfair. This is the story of my first death sentence.

Mr. Albert Lorita was a fifty-four-year-old man who had worked most of his life as a baker. Unmarried and a lifelong resident of New Haven, he was a quiet, simple man, who most enjoyed a game of golf on Saturday followed by a couple of beers. He had always been healthy and had not been in a hospital in his entire life. Late in November, while playing his last round until spring, Mr. Lorita had felt a sharp stabbing pain in his chest after swinging his driver. In a few seconds the pain was gone. Two weeks later he had several similar painful moments on the same day. During the next week the pain came to stay. Several times each hour he felt sharp, knifelike pains that radiated from his back to his abdomen, up into his shoulder, and sometimes into his scrotum. In mid-December he came to the VA clinic. At first the doctors suspected vertebral disease (bits of bone can compress nerve roots and cause substantial pain) and treated him symptomatically, but the pain persisted and worsened. He also began to have difficulty swallowing his food, and he lost his appetite. In early January he underwent a chest x-ray. The results were abnormal, and he was admitted for further studies.

Although one glance at the x-ray raised the possibility of disseminated cancer, no one shared this with Mr. Lorita. One of the ten commandments in medicine is "tissue makes the diagnosis." Until a pathologist had seen a biopsy specimen everybody wanted to give the patient the benefit of the doubt. On the day after Mr. Lorita was admitted to my service, the fellows (doctors taking advanced training) from the various subspecialties were buzzing around his chart like flies. Each was lobbying me in favor of his particular biopsy procedure.

I decided to send Mr. Lorita for a bronchoscopy. This involved a trip to the operating room. A long tube with tiny pincers at its end was put down the throat and into the big airway of a lung. It was then advanced forward until tissue could be bitten off and retrieved. Unfortunately, the bronchoscopy also caused his lung to collapse partially (a pneumothorax is a not uncommon complication, especially when the procedure is done by a new pulmonary fellow). The "pneumo" was not too serious, but it meant that Mr. Lorita would need a chest tube to expand his lung. This, in turn, meant more pain would be added to the symptoms he already had.

Two days later the pathology resident called me to discuss the biopsy report. The news was all bad. Mr. Lorita had metastatic adenocarcinoma. Those bizarre white streaks that I had seen on his x-ray were caused by lymphangitic spread of a cancer. The cancer had begun somewhere outside the lung, at a site where it might even be growing indolently, but it was moving like a wild fire in his chest. The prognosis for a patient whose lungs are full of adenocarcinoma that has spread there from someplace else is extremely grave.

How was I going to dispense this horrible news? I retreated to a bathroom, the only place on the ward where I could find some solitude, and thought the situation over. One thing was clear: Mr. Lorita was going to die, and he was going to die soon. The big question was whether we had anything further to offer him. I knew that the oncologists would want to find out where his cancer had started and to treat him with chemotherapy. I also knew that there was no evidence to show that by identifying the origin of the cancer one could choose a more helpful chemotherapeutic weapon and that there was no evidence that any therapy would help. I made two decisions: First, as he had asked me to, I would tell him the bad news straight without holding out false hopes. Second, I would urge him to refuse invasive, diagnostic studies and try to get him home as soon as possible. Twenty years ago physicians often did not tell patients they had cancer; today they often do. Maybe twenty years from now most physicians will also routinely forego procedures with little benefit so that a dying patient can spend fewer of his last days in a hospital bed.

His sister and aunt were with him, and they agreed to hear the news together. I looked him straight in the eye.

"Mr. Lorita, the news is very bad. You have a cancer that is spread throughout both your lungs. We don't know where it started, but we do know that it started someplace else."

He asked the questions that patients always ask.

"How much time do I have left?"

"Nobody knows, but it won't be long. I would say less than a year, maybe only a few months."

"What happens next?"

"The cancer doctors will probably recommend more tests. They want to find out where the cancer started. Frankly, although they are the experts, I don't think it matters much where your cancer began. I think you should go home as soon as possible to enjoy yourself as much as possible. The cancer doctors will probably recommend a special medicine for you, but you can get it at their clinic." I paused. "Do you have any questions?"

The two women sat silently. He laughed as though I had said something really stupid. Perhaps I had.

"Well, there's nothing more to say, is there? I'm finished. I just want to go home."

"Would you like to see a priest or social worker? Sometimes illness causes a lot of family problems."

"What's a social worker going to do? Hold my hand? No. I don't need them."

"Let me know if you change your mind. I'll see you later today."

The death sentence had only taken a few minutes.

Mr. Lorita took my advice. He refused any further tests. During the week he spent in the hospital (waiting for his pneumothorax to resolve) he became (from the burden of cancer in his lungs) mildly short of breath. When I discharged him I arranged to have an oxygen tank at his home. Just four days later his sister called me. The oxygen seemed to be of little help. He was breathing very fast. I told her to bring him in.

Two hours later I saw him in the emergency room. His face beaded with sweat, he was sitting bolt upright on a stretcher, rapidly gasping huge breaths of pure oxygen through a mask. He looked like a man who had just finished a marathon. I had hardly greeted him before his sister pulled me into the corridor.

"I am praying that he dies tonight," she said.

"Have you talked over how far to go in trying to keep him alive?"

"Yes, he does not want to be put on a respirator."

"OK. Let me just talk privately with him to make sure that he still feels that way. Then I will tell all the other doctors. No one will act against his wishes. He probably will die tonight."

Two tears trickled down her cheeks as she pressed my hands between hers.

"God, I hope he dies this minute."

I stepped inside his cubicle, pulled the green curtains closed, and touched his right arm. Never before or since have I seen a man work so hard to breathe. With each gasp his nostrils flared and his neck muscles stood out. Sweat trickled off his skin, and there was a wild look in his eyes. He stared straight ahead, at first giving no sign of recognition. I squeezed his arm and he turned to me. I spoke.

"Mr. Lorita, I know things are very bad right now, but I have a hard question to ask you. Today could be the end. Your sister says that you do not want to be put on a breathing machine. Is that right?"

The work of breathing precluded speech. He looked squarely at me, nodded affirmatively, and turned away. I stepped out of the room and his crying sister stepped in. It seemed as though he would only be able to sustain his intense activity for a few minutes more. Fighting back my own tears, I sought out the physician in charge of the ER and after explaining the situation, obtained permission to let Mr. Lorita stay where he was rather than transport him upstairs. That done I quietly positioned myself in the hallway opposite his cubicle and waited for his breathing to stop.

Mr. Lorita died two hours later.

Of course there is a lot more to becoming a doctor than learning about death. With time death's drama fades into the background and other moments come forward. When I was a second-year student Dr. Pierre Simon, who introduced my class to clinical medicine, concluded his final lecture with reflections on why it was a privilege to be a physician. He reminded us that for the rest of our lives strangers would disclose to us their most curious and intimate secrets. Despite the hard work, despite the tragedy of many of the stories, how could we not be fascinated and awe-filled by this endless, ever-varying saga of human life? The act of caring for a patient, he promised, was full of subtle but rich rewards. He was right. Let me share some memories I have of my first patients.

I have already mentioned Jack Bodick, the man with end-stage cirrhosis of the liver, who had nearly died from massive bleeding in his gastrointestinal tract. For two weeks he had hovered between life and death in the intensive care unit as the doctors fought to control his bleeding, his metabolic disorders, and a massive pneumonia. Both the physicians and the patient thought that he was going to die. But on the morning that I met him he did not seem to have a care in the world. There was an elfin grin on his gaunt face and a mischievous glint in his Irish eyes. He caught my name tag, and unlike most patients who wait to be spoken to, said, "Hi, Phil. My name's Jack." No need for titles with this guy. He had seen so many young doctors in the last five years that any trace of professional intimidation had long since vanished. I quickly realized that he also knew much more about the management of his disease than did I.

On the second day of my sub, Jack was transferred to a four-bed room on my floor where he stayed for the next six weeks. During that time he taught me a great deal. Taking care of Jack was like driving a truck filled with dynamite; he could explode at any moment. His belly pain could be simple indigestion, but it might also be a peritonitis, the first sign of an impending GI bleed (he also had a duodenal ulcer) or due to an ischemic bowel. About two or three days a week Jack nearly stopped urinating. Oliguria (low urine output) is a serious problem that is managed more by art than by science. Whenever he had not urinated for twelve hours, he generated a maddening amount of scut work for me. But somehow he always started making urine just as I was finishing my workup. About once a week I tapped a liter of fluid from Jack's swollen belly. Although it does not usually work, in theory the act of reducing the volume of fluid in the abdomen will reduce pressure on the vessels to the kidney. The result should be an increase in the perfusion of the kidney, which should make more urine, and hopefully, help to control the ascites. Jack also had chronic anemia, and he "taught" me to follow that closely.

The plan was to get Jack "tuned up" for surgery. There is no good cure for post-cirrhotic ascites. The belly usually stays swollen until death. But an operation called a LeVeen shunt had helped some patients. The process involved putting a tube in the abdomen, running it subcutaneously to the chest, and sewing it into a big vein. The idea was to return the ascitic fluid to the intravascular space so it could be seen by the kidney and excreted. The surgeons wanted to do this procedure, and Jack badly wanted them to try. They visited him daily, to monitor his slow recovery from the GI bleed and to decide when he could become a surgical candidate. Surgeons and internists are trained differently, work differently, and think differently. Hardly a day passed when a surgical resident did not collar me to criticize my management of Mr. Bodick. Being a novice I would listen carefully, and if it made sense, I would take the "advice." A few hours later I would report what I had done to my medical resident, who would promptly "trash" me for doing the wrong thing. After a week or so I stopped taking the surgeons' suggestions. It was much easier to be trashed by them than by my own resident.

Jack taught me that patients can be quite adept at manipulating nurses and doctors. For example, when Jack wanted to get rid of his Cantor tube (a long tube with a weight at the end which is used to manage bowel obstruction) he did not simply yank it out himself or complain bitterly until we removed it. Instead, he drifted steadily downward into a depression. For several days the nurses' notes would chronicle an ever gloomier world view. One morning he would tell me how "down" he felt; that evening he would say that if he could not even drink a cup of juice, there was nothing left to live for. The next day he would tell me that he had decided to commit suicide. Interwoven in these conversations would be occasional references to the tube. For example, he might say, "Look at me. Tubes down my nose and up my penis and an IV line in my arm. Why live?"

When we finally decided to pull the Cantor tube a couple of days earlier than we had planned, Jack's spirits soared. On at least five separate occasions, I saw him go from threats of suicide to optimism in a few hours.

I liked him, but I learned not to trust him. As part of our plan to keep him urinating, we placed him on a low sodium diet (sodium "holds onto" water). Admittedly, this eliminates a lot of tasty foods, but many patients in the hospital easily tolerate this change. One evening I caught Jack with five candy bars, all of which are loaded with sodium. On questioning he admitted that he had paid another patient to go to the canteen, buy the contraband, and slip it to him. After my lecture, he promised not to continue. But the next night I caught him trading food trays with a roommate. He simply could not be trusted. I became almost obsessed with controlling his diet. During meal time I would spy on him. I even took to sneaking into his room at random hours to check on what he was up to. Jack thought this was funny, but it also helped him appreciate that control of his diet was critical. As he became aware of my obsession, his nutritional crimes diminished. In spite of the odds, he slowly improved. He never got well enough to become a surgical candidate, but just as I was completing my subinternship, he left the hospital for a convalescent home.

I remember some patients because of the lessons they taught me about illness and death; I recall other patients because they were great characters. In a hospital noted for its colorful figures, it was, nevertheless, certain that a patient of mine named Joseph Pardis was the most notorious. Pardis (that's what everyone called him) was an old black man who I first met one evening around midnight. He had been shipped in from the worst of the local nursing homes because he was "unresponsive." In fact, he was so profoundly dehydrated that the inside of his mouth was bone dry. When I pulled back the sheet to examine him I immediately thought of the prisoners at Auschwitz. There could not have been more than 120 pounds on his six-foot three-inch frame. I could count every rib in his chest, and when I rolled him over to do a rectal exam his pelvic bones jutted out sharply under his skin.

From the start Pardis made it hard to like him. Although he was moribund, he used his last scrap of strength to fight my exam. Each time that he managed to grab hold of some part of me, I needed to stop and pry myself loose. It was bad enough that I was wrestling with my patient, but he stunk like a dead skunk. Besides his other medical problems Pardis had a history of endocarditis. This meant I had to draw a lot of blood cultures. The blood drawing approximated a gang fight. Two orderlies held him down while I tried to ignore his screams and looked for a decent vein to hit.

Later that night after I finished my arduous workup of Mr. Pardis, I stopped at the nursing station. One of the night nurses asked me about my evening. When I told her about the new arrival, she nearly went into hysterics.

"You mean Pardis is back. I pity you, Doc. That man, he comes in here every six months about to die. A week later he's on his feet, eating double portions, and raising hell. He's one mean dude."

The nurse exactly predicted what would happen. It took us about three days to pour enough fluid into his veins to rehydrate him. During that time his blood cultures grew out *Staphylococcus* bacteria, a finding that earned him a long stay in the hospital to receive IV antibiotic therapy. At rounds when the resident announced this plan, everybody's heart sank. In only three days he had re-established his reputation, and now he would be with us a long time. By only his fifth day on the floor Pardis, who had made a stupendous recovery, was a familiar figure marching up and down the corridors in his ill-fitting unbuttoned green pajamas, dragging his IV pole behind him.

Pardis was not like other patients. As far as he was concerned, the ward was his home and he would do exactly as he pleased. Nurses be damned! He had the bad habit of lying awake moaning most of the night and then sleeping for a good part of the day. He had a particular affection for beds in rooms other than his own. Hardly a day passed when some other patient who had found Pardis asleep in his bed did not plead with me to evict him. Nor did Pardis have any sense of property. Before settling down for a nap in somebody else's bed, he would raid that patient's belongings. He had an incredible appetite and easily demolished many a fellow patient's supply of cookies or candy.

He had one unending complaint about the hospital: We

were trying to starve him! Unlike most people who found the hospital food tepid and tasteless, he loved it. But it came so infrequently and in such small portions! Around six A.M. I usually could find Pardis perched on a chair by the nursing station waiting for breakfast. Our conversation invariably began with his request for the time. After I told him, he would wail bitterly about his hunger pains. About ten days into his hospital course, tired of listening to his observations about the infinitely long wait for breakfast, I produced from my pocket a powdered doughnut and gravely offered it to him. He looked suspiciously at me for a moment, accepted the doughnut, and consumed it in two quick bites. I did not know it, but I had won him over. Never again would he be quite so uncooperative when I tried to draw blood or start an IV.

Pardis had a curious knack for destruction. His single room (no one could stand having him as a roommate) was far messier than any of the rooms with four beds. By dinner time each day it was littered with candy wrappers, crumbs, and dirty pajamas. For reasons known only to him, on the rare occasions when he did sleep in his own bed, he preferred to sleep on the plastic mattress cover, so his sheets were invariably on the floor. About twice a week (for no apparent reason) he ripped his IV line out. Then he casually strolled to the nursing station, a trail of blood marking his path.

During his second week in the hospital, Pardis developed a new habit that was disgusting even by his standards. He had recently started complaining that he could no longer urinate properly. We had worked this problem up as thoroughly as possible, including a urological consult (after which the resident screamed at me for subjecting him to the "Pardis" experience). By all accounts there was nothing wrong with his kidneys or urinary tract, and his complaint that he occasionally "peed in a double-stream" made no sense. Nevertheless, he complained so bitterly that I finally started taking him to the bathroom to watch him urinate—an experience I hope not to repeat.

Quite obviously dissatisfied with our response to his problem, Pardis finally decided to dramatize it. One night about nine o'clock he marched into the nursing station, dropped his drawers, and in full view of myself, an intern and two nurses, peed into the trash bucket. Delighted with the chorus of screams, he announced that his stream was so erratic he needed something as wide as the bucket to pee in. From then on Pardis rarely bothered with bathrooms. There was always a pool of urine by his bedside, and he was frequently sighted peeing in the various trash containers in the hall.

There was only one person in the world to whom Pardis would listen, a sister-in-law named Hattie. She was a poor lady who rode buses for an hour each way to visit him. When Hattie was visiting, Pardis was quiet and cooperative. She was very worried about all the weight he had lost before coming into the hospital. We also feared that his emaciated frame indicated that he had an occult cancer, but Pardis would not consent to any tests. One night, after being chastised by my resident for not getting Pardis to undergo a bone marrow biopsy, I realized that Hattie could make him "consent." I marched into his room with the consent form for the biopsy, explained the test to Hattie, and asked her to persuade him. What I had failed to accomplish in hours of cajoling, she accomplished in five seconds.

"Pardis," she said, "here's a pen. You sign this right now." He meekly complied, and I tried not to think about the ethics of how I obtained his informed consent.

The resident was so frustrated at Pardis's shenanigans that he seemed to delight in doing procedures on him. He was positively eager to supervise my first bone marrow biopsy. But getting a patient to sign a consent form is one thing and convincing him to cooperate with the test is another. As you might have guessed, the bone marrow biopsy did not go smoothly, but it went fast. I had the good sense to premedicate Pardis with an injection of Demerol, but it did not slow him down too much. With the aid of three nurses, we positioned him face down on his bed, cleaned the skin over his iliac crest (back of his hip), and gave him a local anesthetic. As I pricked him with the needle, he started screaming and thrashing, but he could not move. The resident handed me the special, corkscrew-like apparatus used to obtain the sample. Next he literally sat on Pardis's back, and told me to start. I twisted and turned the needle through the skin, muscle, and bone and into the bone marrow as fast as I could, aspirated the spicule-filled marrow, and quickly plunged back in after the bone biopsy. Pardis was screaming his favorite phrase, "I'm hurtin. I'm hurtin." The resident was screaming back at him to shut up. One nurse was laughing, and the other was crying. Pardis had bitten her thumb. The whole procedure took less than five minutes, no doubt the fastest bone marrow biopsy I will ever perform.

For some mysterious reason I actually came to like Pardis. There was an odd humor about him. His behavior was so outrageous that it was funny. Although he nickled and dimed me to death with his litany of needs, most of which he made very late at night, he also put up with a lot from me. Of the fifty or so IV lines that I started in medical school, I probably put one-half into him. Beside the bone marrow biopsy, I also had occasion to tap his knee (which swelled up after he tripped over an IV pole and fell to the floor). From him I learned that with a little work it is possible to establish rapport with nearly every sentient patient, no matter how cantankerous.

Mr. Wilson was my only patient who transcended the land of eccentricity into the world of the truly nuts. He had been admitted to the hospital so we could work up a "coin" lesion in his left lung that had been found accidentally by a routine x-ray. When I went in to do the intake history and physical I strongly suspected that he had lung cancer. It seemed like a straightforward case. We would perform tomograms (special x-rays) of his lungs and a needle biopsy to obtain some tissue for pathological study.

"Good evening, Mr. Wilson. My name is Reilly. [I could not claim the title doctor, but I no longer was willing to admit to being a medical student.] I'll be taking care of you while you are in the hospital. How are you, sir?"

"Fine. I love everybody. Everything's perfect."

I looked a bit closer. He sat on the side of the bed in a bright blue bathrobe and a huge smile. I decided to keep my questions to the point. In response, Mr. Wilson gave me a completely unremarkable history until I asked him if he took any medicines.

"Oh, yeah. My doctor gave me some: lithium syrup, codeine, Seconal, Marplan, and Motrin."

This was a curious list of medicines so I decided to probe further.

"Why Motrin [an anti-inflammatory agent]?"

"Motrin is the key drug. When I take it my world changes. Sometimes I lie in bed at night squeezing my wife's hand for hours while she sleeps. With Motrin the tighter I squeeze the more love I feel flowing between us. It has changed my life. It allows me to express love. For the first time I am able to tell my son that I love him."

"Does Motrin help in other ways?" I asked.

"At night I can see snowstorms that are not really there."

After I had finished the history and physical exam, a period marked by several exclamations by my new patient that he loved me and the hospital, I talked to Mr. Wilson about his upcoming tests. I explained the purpose of taking the special x-rays and doing a needle biopsy of his lung. He was completely indifferent and unworried.

"I am not scared. God loves me and His will be done."

I did not know if Mr. Wilson suffered from a manic-depressive illness, or schizophrenia, and I did not care. I just wanted him to remain stable. I had enough trouble dealing with Pardis and Bodick.

The first problem with Mr. Wilson's stay in the hospital began when my resident told me to stop the Motrin because there was no clear indication for it. When he discovered this change, Mr. Wilson cried inconsolably.

When I tried to reason with him, things got worse.

"The Motrin does nothing but good things," he insisted. "I would rather stop all my other medicines."

I made a decision. "Mr. Wilson, let's make a pact. You can take all that Motrin you brought with you into the hospital, but we won't give you any new pills. But, don't tell anybody I told you to do this, OK?" That was fine with him.

For the rest of the week Mr. Wilson was fine. The needle biopsy was delayed over the weekend, so he roamed the halls, visiting other patients and befriending everyone. Everytime he saw me he pulled me aside to tell me how "beautiful" he found the hospital.

"You're all beautiful, all the lovely nurses and handsome young doctors. And you all work so hard for everyone."

He had clearly been watching too much television. The last I saw of Mr. Wilson he was lying in bed smiling broadly, totally unconcerned that the biopsy was positive for cancer and that he had to undergo major surgery.

During my sub I drew blood at least two hundred times, punctured the radial artery to obtain "ABGs" (arterial blood gases) about twenty times, and tapped fluid from human chests, abdomens, and knees. By the end of the six weeks I had become downright cocky about my prowess with a needle, delighting in the challenge of "drawing" someone whose veins had stymied other phlebotomists. In lighter moments I reflected that in exchange for fifty thousand dollars and four years of my life, Yale had made me one of the best blood-drawing technicians in the nation. In six weeks I performed gram stains on dozens of samples of human sputum, urine, and joint fluid. With time my total bewilderment gradually gave way to rudimentary diagnostic skill. My eyes grew sufficiently used to the strange microscopic world of delicate pink rods and richly purple clumps of cocci that I became able to correlate their presence with the various pneumonias from which my patients suffered. I marveled at the power of these tiny organisms and was awestruck by the even greater power of the drugs that killed them. I listened to the beat of innumerable hearts and issued hundreds of commands "to breathe slowly in and out through your mouth." Words like *rales, rhonchi, crackles,* and *wheezes* finally began to take on meaning, as the necessary neural roads were paved between the auditory centers and the memory cells of my brain. I still was at the beginning, but I had made a start.

I also learned one great fact about clinical medicine: It is dirty, hard work, much more akin to construction work or waitressing than being a lawyer or banker.

The diagnostic lessons were often learned painfully. One day at rounds after I had described my physical exam of a patient, the attending physician yelled "catch," and threw a rubber glove at me.

"Go feel the left axilla again," he said, implying that I had missed an enlarged lymph node.

When I re-examined the patient, repeatedly digging deeply into his armpit, I finally found a pea-sized node that I had not felt before. I felt a wincing embarrassment that morning, but I probably will not miss too many axillary lymph nodes in my life.

I often wonder why clinicians sometimes teach by ridicule. True, most of us remember facts tied to such moments. But surely the repeated bruising of the ego must have a harmful effect on a young physician. Is it possible that one becomes driven more by fear of ridicule than by a desire to help the patient? Of course, the counter argument is that the end justifies the means. The important thing is that one does a thorough physical examination. But I have a nagging fear that when our errors are ridiculed, however well-intentioned, we begin to hate the patients who "tricked" us as well as the doctors who were more clever.

Despite my criticism of the manner in which it was sometimes taught, the single most important lesson I learned during my subinternship was the principle of thoroughness. It was a lesson that was taught every day in myriad ways by the nurses, the house staff, and the patients themselves. I learned it from the nurses with whom I "hung" blood. They were exquisitely careful in matching the patient's wrist band number to the sequence printed on the bag of packed cells which we were about to pour into his veins. I learned it from the interns, who, having been "burned" countless times, would not let me sign out my patients without challenging my assertions that there was no acute problems. Over and over again patients taught me that in real people disease does not behave in the way proclaimed by textbooks. Most of all, I learned to be thorough from a senior resident named David File.

For the last four weeks of my sub, David was the team leader. An ex-college basketball player, his six-foot two-inch frame was accentuated by trousers with a military crease and a ramrod posture. Even among a crew of very bright house officers, David's command of medical literature was awesome. He seemed better read than most of the attendings. He had excellent recall and a real interest in teaching, so if I stayed alert, not a moment of rounds was wasted.

I do not know if he loved clinical medicine, but I am

certain that David had an unmatched commitment to help people get better. For him every sick patient was a challenge, and he definitely liked to win. One day while we were talking in the ICU, David heard a patient (for whom our team was not caring) with a nonproductive pneumonia finally "york up" some phlegm. In a flash he grabbed a sputum cup and captured the sample, asking me to gram stain it. I agreed, but turning back to the problem we were discussing, it slipped from my mind. The next day at rounds when we walked past the patient who had coughed, David, who had been up all night and seen a dozen other patients, remembered to ask me about the gram stain. I confessed failing to do it and felt horrible when he looked me squarely in the eye and said, "We're slipping, we let the patient down." He meant it.

David had the enviable ability to integrate the human and the scientific aspects of clinical medicine. He once helped me take care of a man with an unusually slow heartbeat, a condition which frequently made him dizzy and threatened sudden death. David spent an entire afternoon teaching me about sick sinus syndrome. He delighted in hooking the man up to an EKG machine and instructing him to perform various physical maneuvers that might change his heart rate. He even had me inject a test dose of a drug called atropine to see if it would override the *bradycardia* and speed up his heart. Dave also spent several hours trying to convince this man, whose heart rate sometimes dropped as low as 30, that he needed a pacemaker, but he did not succeed.

Dave and I also took care of a fragile oldtimer named Mr. August Dillon. Well over eighty and burdened with multiple medical problems, the worst of which was a worn out heart muscle, Mr. Dillon was the kind of patient many house officers hated to have on service. At any minute anything could go wrong, and the closer one looked, the more trouble one found. Many residents preferred not to look too closely or come too quickly if trouble started. Not David. Every single day before we left the hospital he huddled with me to review Mr. Dillon's tortoiselike progress. How did he look? Was he moving from bed to chair (he was on a cardiac rehabilitation program)? What did the afternoon EKG show (I was getting twice-daily electrocardiograms because he had an unusual rhythm)? What was his digoxin level (the blood level of this heart medicine had gotten too high because his kidneys were not eliminating it)? How in the world did Dave find time to do this with two or three of my patients as well as with the other subs' and carry out all his other tasks? It was beyond me. Many times as Paul and I walked down the cinder block stairs to the freedom of an evening at home, we marveled at "Superman," as we had privately nicknamed him.

Another lesson I learned during my sub was the principle of distance. Much as a young physician would like to bathe his patients in compassion, it simply is not possible. The patients are too sick, there are too many of them, and the doctor is too busy or too tired. I had heard this line of argument before my sub, but I had never quite believed it. Doctors today, I argued, fancy themselves scientists, not healers. They are clinically myopic, seeing only the diseased organ, not the whole person. Their technological powers have turned their heads. As they spend more time reading journal articles and consulting subspecialists about the results of esoteric tests, they spend less time at the patient's bedside. Indeed, at times the house staff seemed to place a higher priority on having third-year students chase down laboratory data than on having them examine a patient. I was frequently told to "run down to nuclear medicine," but rarely asked "to go talk to Mr. Jones." I still wonder if the power of doctors to diagnose and cure has sapped their power to care.

If that is, in fact, the case, it is not without reason. The "system," which controls the way that doctors must work in hospitals, does not permit much time or energy to be devoted to the task of caring. If you acquiesce to the system, your time is spent gathering data. Medical care is premised on the accumulation of facts. The house officer must spend time scheduling tests, drawing blood, carrying specimens to the lab, and pondering an ever-growing mass of data. Indeed, we draw so much blood from patients for laboratory study that our major therapeutic maneuver may match that of the late eighteenth century. Then physicians applied leeches; today we use butterflies (the name for the small needles used to get in the veins of many old folks)! A physician responsible for the diagnostic workup of a dozen patients has little time left for talking with or comforting them. After all, a physician who does not properly manage the case may harm the patient. The fact is that most patients would probably choose a technically superior physician over a more compassionate, but less skilled, colleague.

The only way I could reasonably cope with this dilemma was to adjust my expectations. I began a relationship with a patient, knowing I would probably not get to know him or her very well. At the outset I always tried to explain this and to help the patient understand why it was so; gradually, I realized that it was unnecessary. At a teaching hospital the patient is overwhelmed with visits from doctors, medical students, interns, residents, and attendings who parade to the bedside and gravely ask after his or her health while they think of technical issues. The sheer mass of white coats usually generates the illusion of concern. For most patients that is acceptable. Indeed, I even had patients rebuff my efforts to get to know them. They were tired of visits from doctors and nurses, and they wanted to watch reruns of "M.A.S.H."

But there was more to the principle of distance than dealing with one's sense of obligation. There was the problem of pain, or revulsion, or horror. Call it what you

will. On a medicine service the diagnostic skills of physicians eclipse their therapeutic powers. Patients often have
chronic or incurable illness against the progression of
which our therapeutic skills are woefully weak. When
cancer is dancing through someone's body, or a dried out,
gnarled liver, or a floppy heart muscle, or a stroked-out
brain prevails, there is little that a doctor can offer. The
patient abhors learning this, and the doctor abhors admitting it. At times they both feel completely impotent. There
is one great difference between them. For better or worse,
patients live out their life, incorporating the disease into it
and dealing with it as best they can. Doctors repeatedly
recognize their impotence. It becomes part of their life
rhythm. How odd to be endowed with power by others,
yet to feel so powerless inside.

Inevitably, indeed very quickly, one begins to separate
oneself from the whole business. The doctor delivers the
news, be it good or bad, succinctly and honestly, trying not
to embellish the facts with too many false hopes. Compassion is limited to minutes, while the statement "I'm very
sorry" is again repeated. Then the doctor flees, leaving
behind the bad news, another glaring reminder of such
powerlessness.

Beside giving bad news, the doctor must contend with
the decrepitude of age, the cruelty of stroke and senility,
and the great inequity of cancer. On our ward there was a
saying about any new patient that we liked: "He's a good
guy. He must have cancer." How long can one walk
through such a world without developing a thick emotional
callus? If the pain gets too great, is it not natural to back
away from it just as you back away from a hot oven? For
each new patient requiring care, the physician unconsciously draws some emotional perimeter to define the
interaction. The dimensions vary tremendously. I was one
of the few people who were willing to visit Mr. Garabedian. On the other hand, I remember a man whose cancer

had invaded his spinal cord. He lay on a metal frame in the intensive care unit, paralyzed from the neck down, fully conscious, waiting to die. I could not bear to look at him. I hated even to think about his illness. He transcended compassion. It was too horrible, and I avoided him and rejoiced when he died.

Sometimes I fantasize that patients with chronic disease struggle with their doctors in the same way that drowning men grapple with their saviors. Some secret force drives the drowning man to take the other swimmer down. Did patients to whom I got too close infect me with their illness, their rage, their foreboding of death? How could I help but hate them for it? Why was it that I heard so many young doctors vow to commit suicide rather than linger in chronic illness on a hospital ward? This is a tragic paradox. For they are rejecting the very treatment options that society rewards them handsomely for offering to others. If house officers routinely articulate this opinion, that death is preferable to chronic care in a hospital, surely there is something very wrong with the way that care is delivered. Recently, a nonphysician told me that his greatest fear in getting old was "becoming dehumanized" by doctors. He complained that the powers that be seem to pay little attention to the aspects of hospital care that cause feelings of dehumanization. He wondered, "Do physicians go to different hospitals than the lay public or are they more emotionally resilient?" The answer is of course no, physicians are not more resilient; they have learned the principle of distance and applied it even to themselves.

Another lesson that I learned during my subinternship was that the realities of scientific discovery engender a clinical enthusiasm that is illusionary. This is a most controversial assertion, but I believe that it is true. Professors of medicine delight in stating that "the corpus of biomedical knowledge is doubling every five years," or "after your senior year of residency your competence as a physician begins to decline" (because you move away from the centers of learning), or "patient care changes so radically that it is impossible for any doctor to stay up in all but the most narrowly defined field." Of course we are in the midst of a knowledge explosion that seems unending. Subspecialties are proliferating at an incredible pace. There are diagnostic radiologists, therapeutic radiologists, pediatric radiologists, and bone radiologists. Internal medicine has spawned endocrinologists, who in turn have spawned diabetologists. Amidst all these incredible developments, what has happened to the common patients with the common illnesses? How dramatically have their treatments changed?

One evening not long after finishing my subinternship I tried to get a handle on this question by asking two physicians who had been interns thirty years ago to explain how they had managed two problems that I had seen: pulmonary embolism and uncomplicated myocardial infarction. "When we suspected a PE," said one, "we put the patient to bed and started an intravenous line and gave heparin. We kept him for about ten days." I was surprised. He had just described the basics of our treatment protocol. There were differences. In the fifties various lab tests to study blood clotting parameters were not as readily available and the heparin could not be so uniformly delivered. But as we talked more I began to suspect that the mortality from pulmonary embolism has probably not changed significantly. The management of heart attacks, on the other hand, seems to have changed dramatically in the last twenty-five years. Nearly every urban hospital now has a coronary care unit. There are wonderful new drugs to reduce the heart's workload and mechanical aids like the "balloon" (a counter-pulsation device to assist the heart's delivery of blood to the body). But, in 1951, a "simple" MI was managed with bed rest, oxygen, and morphine, just as it is today. And for all our efforts survival from an uncomplicated heart attack has not changed all that much since my older physician friend stalked the halls of his hospital thirty-five years ago.

Do scientific advances breed a false certainty, causing the doctor to discount the basics of bedside medicine and to shift focus from the patient's face to the computer printout? I don't know. But if an expanding knowledge base diminishes contact with patients, there must be some downside to the scientization of medicine. I particularly worry about the art of clinical medicine. I finished my subinternship still romantically committed to the classic image of the physician—a concerned person with special knowledge committed to helping his fellow man. Perhaps no physician can be taught how to care, but medical schools need always to try.

Chapter 9

THE MATCH

Everyone thinks that medical school is a four-year program, but in fact it is virtually over at the end of the third-year clinical clerkships. Although there are huge gaps in medical students' knowledge and an infinite number of "electives" (brief periods during which a student may study specific kinds of illness, such as kidney diseases) offer a chance to fill them, their minds are elsewhere. During the summer and autumn of the fourth year, they are lame ducks, obsessively preoccupied with two questions: What field should I choose? Where should I apply? As the student ponders these questions, everything else—senior thesis, the renal elective, learning to read EKGs—becomes little more than a perfunctory chore. The real mental juices flow only when they think about the future.

The uninitiated may wonder: "Why so much fuss about choosing a specialty? After all, a doctor is a doctor. They all see patients and they all own sailboats." But doctors don't all see patients, and they don't all own sailboats. In fact, the differences among certain medical specialties may be greater than the differences between being a doctor and a lawyer or an engineer. A therapeutic radiologist may devote much time to problems of high-energy physics. His reading will often focus on epidemiology and statistics; he wants to see the numbers to prove that a new therapy is actually extending the lives of patients afflicted with certain kinds of cancer. Contrary to your visions of the autopsy table, the majority of a pathologist's career may be spent in a spanking clean laboratory not unlike the work places of thousands of scientists and technicians. A psychiatrist is likely to work in a comfortable sitting room talking with patients about their problems. Such work is more akin to that of a "trusts and estates" attorney than to that of a neurosurgeon, who may start the hospital day before dawn and spend eight hours behind an operating microscope removing a brain tumor. The obstetrician is never able to predict which night will be spent lying on a hospital cot waiting for a baby, while the ENT (ear, nose, and throat) surgeon rarely gets called out at odd hours. One could go on and on.

In addition to training one in the basic facts of medicine, the multiplicity of third-year clerkships was intended to show us our career options. But the clerkships demand so much time and energy that it is difficult for medical students to step back from the trees and see the forest. There is little opportunity to ruminate. After completing an internal medicine clerkship on Friday afternoon, one has two days to sleep before plunging into surgical training at six o'clock on Monday morning. Every six weeks, students confront unfamiliar faces, are challenged with questions they cannot answer, and are asked to do things they have never thought of doing before. There is no time to think about the prior clerkship, and if, several weeks after being immersed in the current rotation, one does try to recall the past, it seems a million years ago. No wonder so many medical students feel unprepared to choose a residency!

The major challenge of the clerkship is to learn the diagnosis and therapy of the illnesses from the patients that one's team follows. But a tremendous amount of psychic energy is expended on another critically important task. Clinical clerks have to quickly assess their residents, to learn what they expect, and to decide whether they are friendly, good teachers or aloof tyrants who might harm them irreparably with their written evaluations. This task is exacerbated by the fact that both the interns and the residents frequently rotate off service during the clerks' six-week stay. The clerks must evaluate the new team members, all the time worrying that they will not be interested in teaching or that they will expect a style of behavior totally different from the last residents. This can range from trivial to crucial subjects. For example I started one clerkship with a resident who told me not to wear a necktie; two weeks later a new resident asked me why I was not wearing one. More importantly, the first resident refused to let me do procedures like thoracenteses or placement of central lines; his successor was critical of me for not knowing how to perform the same operations. But he thoroughly instructed me in these techniques.

The parade of house officers complicates clinical clerks' ability to reach conclusions about the specialties through which they rotate. The personality and style of each resident, as well as of the other team members, shapes one's image of the specialty. I looked forward to my clerkship in general surgery, a specialty I was considering as a career choice, but the chief resident at the community hospital in which I trained was so unfriendly and unwilling to teach that he soured me on the field. To the outsider this may seem foolish. Why let one bad experience change your interests? Remember, though, it is also your *only* clinical experience in the specialty. When some resident has given you a hard time beginning at six A.M. every day for six weeks, it is horrible to imagine continuing that for two or three years. Like it or not, the clerkship experience varies tremendously depending on the idiosyncracies of the house staff and, of course, the third-year students themselves. It is mostly a question of luck, yet your future will be shaped by those ineffable forces.

Even if each clerkship went smoothly, medical students still face a difficult choice. First of all, there are vast areas of medicine to which they may not be formally exposed during the third year. This includes radiology, dermatology, and ophthalmology. In other fields the exposure is very brief. For example, my official training in anesthesiology took place on three mornings of my surgical clerkship. I started a few intravenous lines, intubated one patient, and "bag-breathed" a man through a cholecystectomy. Of course, I was indirectly exposed to anesthesiology throughout my surgical clerkship, but there is little contact between the person holding the retractors and the person "passing gas" behind the curtain that separates the anesthesiologist from the surgical field.

During the fourth year, students may take electives in specialty fields. But there are competing demands for their time. Many students, eager to secure another good letter of recommendation, devote the summer of the fourth year to doing subinternship. Preparation of a thesis frequently requires several months. A few students did most of the research during the summer after their first year, but most of us procrastinated, and the fourth year was the next block of available time.

Except for about twenty people whom God blessed with certainty as to career choice (people who started medical school *knowing* they would become psychiatrists, ophthalmologists, or orthopedic surgeons), most of my classmates and I lost a lot of sleep trying to choose a residency. Talking scores of times with dozens of medical students, I found that we tended to weigh the demands of the residency only slightly less than the nature of the practice that we would enter after we completed training. After countless hours of thinking, I realized that choosing a residency represented the first major branch point for most medical students in their adult lives. For a minimum of seven years, four years in college followed by three years in medical school, they had been working a lot harder and having a lot less fun than most people who had not chosen to go into medicine. Their college friends had already graduated from law school. Some of them were now working for big New York firms making impressive salaries—with *no* night call! Many college friends were starting to raise families, but only a fraction of my class had married, and hardly any had children. For many med students choosing a residency loomed as a decision about lifestyle. This was a crucial opportunity to reorder their priorities. Childhood dreams of oneself as the tireless young physician now faced competition with visions of a cheese omelet, Mozart, and the *New York Times* in a cozy bedroom on a Sunday morning.

Although there were many others as well, I heard my classmates ask six major questions when thinking about a specialty choice: What will the patients be like? How many years is the training? What is the call schedule? How are the hours? How crowded is the field? How lucrative is it?

From the medical students' perspective there is a huge difference between a surgical residency that runs five to six years with four years of heavy night call (remaining awake in the hospital) and a medical residency, which lasts three years with only two years of heavy night call. Surgeons usually start work at six A.M., while internists may start as "late" as seven-thirty in the morning. As one resident once said to me, "You've got to *love* the operating room. Given the choice, you have to want it more than a vacation in the Virgin Islands or a weekend with a beautiful blonde. If you don't want it that badly, don't go into surgery." Given that surgery and its subspecialties are overcrowded, newly trained surgeons probably will not have the power to choose where they will work. They may never match the income earned by older colleagues—a critical fact in a world that operates on the principle of delayed gratification. I definitely preferred the glamor of the OR and the surgeon's ability to make people well over the stale odors of the medical ward and the frustrations felt by the internist managing patients with incurable illness. But as one of my classmates who very much wanted to become a surgeon put it, "Five years of your life is a heavy price to pay for the right to cut on bowels." He was right. When push came to shove, I knew that I couldn't hack the training.

Of course, each student sees the choice from a different vantage point. After she hit the wards, Pat, a sensitive, caring woman who came to medical school intending to go into pediatrics, simply could not accept the time commitment demanded by that residency. She felt that it would eliminate any chance of marriage and children before she reached her thirties. In the end she chose to take a radiology residency in a large city. Training in radiology has relatively normal-looking hours with little night call. She would be working eight to five just like the rest of America, and she would be entering a field in which she would combine being a parent and a professional with roughly the same difficulties faced by women in law and business.

Another big question was to determine what kinds of patients we most enjoyed. There are really three questions here: What patients do I most enjoy? What problems do I find most interesting? What procedures (if any) do I prefer?

Internal medicine, the largest specialty in the profession, is becoming "geriatric" medicine. An internist sees few patients under forty, and many patients are over sixty-five. It is not uncommon to devote a major portion of time to the care of nursing home patients. When they rotate through internal medicine, students tend to see the oldest, sickest persons in the society. The patients may be querulous, senile, uncooperative, and combative. Frankly, one gets little pleasure from examining the body of a decrepit, old stroke patient. Pediatrics is a sharp contrast. Some students infinitely prefer the "well-child" exam, a key element of general pediatrics, to doing a "routine physical" on a seventy-five-year-old diabetic patient. The child is soft, smooth, and supple. Even the sickest children often have beautiful bodies. As one otherwise very compassionate classmate put it, "I just can't stand doing rectal exams on 'gomes' (none too affectionate slang for oldtimers with chronic disease). Give me the screaming two-year-old any day." On the other hand, some of us had little tolerance for wrestling with two-year-olds or being sprayed with urine by infants.

In deciding which work we would find most enjoyable, it was important to imagine the never-never land beyond residency. In the "tertiary care" centers at which most of us would train, the patients would all have complicated illnesses. Otherwise they would not be there. But when we thought about private practice (with which we had *no* experience), the three major specialties devoted to patient care seemed very different. General pediatrics is an office practice. A lot of energy is devoted to following the development of well children, to educating their parents, and to practicing preventive medicine. One of the doctors who taught me pediatrics told me that he had not had a patient die in twenty-five years. Naturally, some students are drawn to general pediatrics because its happy, upbeat nature more than compensates for its *relative* lack of diagnostic challenge. Pediatrics is fun.

A general surgeon sees patients of all ages (the thirteen-year-old boy with appendicitis, the forty-six-year-old woman with gallbladder disease, and the sixty-seven-year-old man with bowel cancer) who are often healthy with the exception of one problem—hopefully, a problem that can be fixed. Further, the surgeon has the incomparable pleasure derived from making sick people become well, as anyone who has been doubled over by a hot appendix knows. The surgeon acts, knows what has to be done and does it. Some students find this tremendously attractive. Other students, perhaps after holding retractors on their fifth cholecystectomy, begin to think that surgery demands all brawn and no brains. In medical school the great emphasis is on diagnosis and it is internal medicine, not surgery, that reigns supreme in that art. But uncommon diseases happen uncommonly, and the vast majority of patients seen by an internist do not present major diagnostic challenges. I remember how my heart sank when an internist, whom I asked to describe his practice, said that he spent 70 percent of his time managing hypertension. Some of my classmates worried that "internists pushed pills" for a living.

Some medical students are so attracted or repelled by procedures that their careers are shaped by this consideration alone. Pediatricians have one great art to master: drawing blood and starting intravenous lines on the tiny vessels of infants. They also do a few spinal taps, but these are actually quite easy on children. Except for those who specialize in intensive care, most pediatricians don't often do procedures. This is one reason why they make significantly less money than other doctors. The fee structures of insurance companies are keyed to what a doctor does to a patient, not the time spent. Internists do a fairly broad array of minor procedures: spinal taps, arterial blood gases, paracenteses, placement of central lines, sigmoidoscopies, and bone marrow biopsies. If they go into a subspecialty, especially cardiology or gastroenterology, their practices may become very "procedure oriented," and their incomes may soar. "Invasive cardiologists" spend their mornings in the "cath lab," gowned like surgeons and armed with their tools, as they run long catheters from "cut down" sites in the arm or leg into the heart. Of course, surgeons are the masters of procedures. Indeed, that is what dominates their lives. They are the ones who venture into the hidden places, never sure of what they will find, knowing they must meet whatever challenge they uncover. Some medical students hate the world of knives and needles and

M.A.S.H. mentality; others love it. And they find their niche.

Although I cannot for the life of me figure out how we did it, in the autumn of our senior year we all made the choice: medicine, pediatrics, surgery, psychiatry, radiology—whatever it was. For many of us choosing a residency seemed to be made on the basis of which field had the fewest drawbacks. It was a process of elimination. In describing how this is done, I can only speak for myself, but I think that others had similar experiences.

There were two specialties that I excluded quite early from consideration. Obstetrics was completely out. I had been very impressed by seeing how frequently forty-five-year-old obstetricians spent their nights sleeping on army cots in a dingy call room waiting to deliver babies who rarely needed assistance in making their entry. I had also spent a week observing an obstetrician at work in his office. It seemed that he did little more than take out IUDs, measure swelling bellies, and draw blood. True, obstetrics and gynecology is a happy specialty (assuming one avoids the care of patients with cancers) that may be quite lucrative. But in practice it seemed intellectually barren, the hours are horrible, and the cloud of malpractice darkens it.

For very different reasons I decided early that I would not become a psychiatrist. Psychiatry is attractive in many ways. It is fascinating to work with acutely ill patients with whom you can travel to the inner reaches of the mind. The field is deeply intellectual. To a good psychiatrist every corner of the realm of human experience—art, music, ethnography, animal behavior and children at play—beckons as a source of learning. Further, psychiatry is on the brink of a biochemical revolution that will reshape the therapeutic approach to people suffering from schizophrenia and endogenous depression. But academic psychiatry, the world in which one may participate in and appreciate efforts to understand the psychology of artistic creation or the biochemistry of depression, is vastly different from private practice. Most psychiatrists make their livings by listening to members of the middle class work through their neuroses or deal with alcohol abuse. I doubted that such people were "sick" and knew that psychiatrists had little ability to make them "well." At the risk of sounding harsh, many therapeutic encounters reminded me too much of an adult baby-sitting service. To be a psychiatrist you have to believe in the therapeutic value of a certain kind of intellectual exercise; I did not.

I daydreamed frequently about becoming a surgeon. No medical student who has watched a resident "crack" a chest to set up a "triple" (coronary artery bypass graft) for an attending has not succumbed at least once to this fantasy. I still vividly recall one night in the ER, when a man was brought in with four bullets in his chest. As a dozen nurses and residents worked frantically over him in the trauma room, the thoracic surgeon stood in the doorway calmly surveying the scene before going to the OR. In a few minutes he would slit this man wide open, go after the bullets, stop the bleeding, and save his life. What power! But the training by which one acquires it is grueling, and the responsibility one must shoulder is weighty. During the clerkship year I realized that I did not have the desire or the stamina to fulfill my fantasy.

By August of my fourth year I had narrowed my choice to pediatrics or medicine. Because I was fascinated with the problems of genetic disease, a subspecialty in pediatrics, I preferred academic pediatrics to medicine. Pediatricians also seemed friendlier and less competitive than their counterparts in the medical program. But I did not envision an academic career, and private pediatricians care for few children with genetic diseases. They refer them to specialty clinics. I agreed that the work done by community pediatricians—the careful observation of a child's development, attention to the details of preventive medicine such as immunization and the use of car seats for infants—was crucial, but it did not excite me.

Largely by a process of elimination and not without misgiving, I chose to seek an internship in internal medicine. In making this choice I was troubled by two perceptions. First, because internists take care of old people, they are frequently charged with managing the decline and demise of their patients, whereas surgeons, after finishing their work or deciding they have nothing to offer, return their patients to the care of internists. Second, many of the patients for whom internists care, especially during their residency, are chronically and incurably ill because of self-abuse. They have destroyed their livers with alcohol and their lungs with cigarettes. They suffer from endocarditis because of heroin addiction. Frankly, most alcoholics and drug addicts do not elicit that sense of compassion that a physician wants to feel. But it is also the internist who is most frequently challenged by diagnostic problems and most directly confronted by the mysteries of disease. There is something compelling about disease. One may appreciate a rare ailment just as an art lover savors a Breughel or a Bosch; it is beautiful in part because it is beyond understanding. Internal medicine is also the broadest field that one can choose to train in. One can go in more directions with it when one is done.

After choosing a field, the next step is to secure the appropriate forms and apply for residency programs. But medical students' ignorance about training programs (except for those directly associated with their school) is even greater than their ignorance of the field. How then were my colleagues and I to choose where to apply? Beside countless conversations in which students and house officers trade unreliable opinions about various programs, fourth-year students may turn to the few attending clinicians they have gotten to know (for advice that may be no more reliable) and the chairman of the specialty which they plan to enter. At Yale they also must visit the dean of students, ostensibly to receive some sage advice on this subject.

I arrived for my appointment with the chief of the Department of Internal Medicine in a pessimistic mood. The few classmates who had mentioned their interviews had uniformly characterized them as humbling—in keeping with the rest of medical school. It was twenty minutes after the hour (and the next student had already arrived for his interview) before the chief summoned me. By the time I made it to the chair in front of his desk he was on the telephone. The next fifteen minutes were terrible. As I tried to tell him a little bit about myself and get his opinions about various programs, the phone was ringing as though we were in a precinct station. He kept taking the calls. By the fifth interruption, I decided that he had no interest in helping me, and I definitely had no desire to talk to him. Maybe he read the anger in my face, because he finally told his secretary to hold his calls. Already doomed, our interview began.

I knew that my evaluations placed me in the upper portion of the class, although certainly not at the top. I also knew that I wanted to move on for my residency.

"Assuming I do not wish to apply to Yale," I asked, "where would you recommend?"

Glancing up from my folder, he launched into the usual generalities.

"Forget about the Brigham and the General because you won't get in. You have a shot everywhere else. Don't go to Columbia [currently, there was bad blood between the departments of medicine at the two schools]. Penn, Rochester, Cornell . . . they are all very good." The conversation continued in this way for another five or six minutes. The last twenty minutes had taken their toll. The next time the phone rang I decided to leave rather than waiting to be dismissed. His eyebrows raised ever so slightly as I politely nodded and quickly departed.

My interview with the dean of students did not fare much better. It was a visit that he required before writing the "dean's letter" that Yale sent out in lieu of a transcript. (One consequence of the Yale "system" was that with no grades to review, it was difficult for others to assess our performance.) Save for the handful of exceptionally successful or unusually unsuccessful students, these letters were rumored to be barely distinguishable from each other. Because of their similarity, most of us guessed that these missives were much less important than the letters written by attendings, the physicians who were responsible for overseeing the ward teams.

Some of my classmates were quite critical about the value of the interview. One woman who had asked for advice about programs in obstetrics, a field that Yale students are not encouraged (except by obstetricians) to enter, complained that she had gotten a brushoff. Another friend said, "Expect five minutes on your folders, five minutes on your list (of programs), and five minutes of the dean's trivia." He called it perfectly. The only thing I remember about the interview was that after telling him I might apply for a residency at the Dartmouth program, the dean, a friendly fellow, told me he had once played the piano at the Dartmouth Inn. So it goes.

Most hospitals require that their intern applicants supply at least two letters of recommendation from physicians who have observed them working with patients in the specialty that they have decided to pursue. For each clinical clerkship an attending is "on service." He or she supervises the resident who leads the house officer team and is ultimately responsible for the care that all the patients receive. It is also the attending's duty to teach the house officers and the medical students. Medical students "present" their patients to the attending, discussing the differential diagnosis and the therapeutic plan.

From the students' perspective this system leaves little room to maneuver. They are assured of getting to know at least one or, in the case of internal medicine, two attendings well enough to ask them to write on their behalf. But if the student and the attending do not "click," or if the student really does a poor job, there is a problem. For the attending's letter is crucial to "matching" in a top residency. This is especially true at schools where students are not graded and no class rank is compiled.

Fortunately, we were permitted to review our clerkship evaluations. This permits students to make a pretty good guess about the kind of letter that would be written on their behalf. In extreme cases this calculation may generate major career changes. One of my classmates, an extraordinarily hard working, intelligent, and sensitive guy—easily one of our best students—had the bad luck of drawing two attendings in internal medicine who just did not like his style. He very much wanted a career in academic medicine but he knew he could not get recommendations that would guarantee him a slot in what he called the "big time." At the last minute he switched his residency choice from medicine to pediatrics, a field in which he could get strong letters. He was admitted to one of the top pediatric programs in the country.

I had a fairly typical experience in securing my letters of recommendation. Having chosen internal medicine, and having scheduled my subinternship sufficiently late that my performance would not be a factor in my residency application, I turned to the two attendings who had been my perceptors during third year. On first medicine I had drawn a young, affable physician who had written a glowing evaluation, probably better than I deserved and certainly as superlative as anyone could want. On second medicine I had been evaluated by a senior faculty member, a leading clinician, but a laconic, reserved man whom I had not impressed. I knew that in his mind I was competent, but definitely not "great." Given the interactions we had had, I considered his evaluation to be fair. There were no sour grapes. I had received excellent evaluations in all clerkships except "second medicine." Coming out of Yale, this meant that I had a reasonable shot at getting admitted to a leading residency program. I was pretty sure that I did not want to stay at Yale. After five years in New Haven I was tired of pizza (the city's major cuisine), "old blues," and the ugly statue on top of East Rock that seemed to monitor every move I made. I was ready to move on.

I wanted to train in Boston. The decision to put the geographic factor ahead of *all* others in choosing a residency was a major change in "career" planning. It was also not compatible with the assumption at Yale that one should always go to the most prestigious program possible. Both the dean and my attendings were gently, but unquestionably, critical of my original plan to apply only to Boston programs. Knowing that I had only a fair chance at being accepted to the Harvard programs, but a good shot at top programs in Philadelphia or New York, they urged me to be a little less inflexible. Eventually, I caved in and applied to two programs in New York and the one at Dartmouth.

Despite my critics, I felt my concern for geography was reasonable. In general, most medical students plan their residencies around the concept of the "big name." But a famous program is not necessarily the best program in which to train. In more than a few cases the "name" had long survived the circumstances that generated its reputation. Some of the top programs were known to treat their interns much worse than did other, only slightly less prestigious programs. They demanded more nights on call in exchange for less money and the risk of receiving more psychic abuse. Other top residency programs involved much time caring for the patients admitted by private practitioners—people who can make an intern's life somewhat less comfortable than six months in Hell. Since the "best" internship is a harsh experience, it seemed to me that the best strategy was to protect oneself as much as possible. There were only two ways to do that: Pick a city in which you will enjoy living for three to five years, and choose a program that promised to hurt you a little less than the others. Given that prospects for a career in academic medicine were determined more by one's fellowship work than one's residency, my logic seemed impeccable—to me at least.

Many of my classmates did not agree. I wound up filing the initial application forms with ten programs in the New York–Boston area. Most of the seniors filed far more than ten to institutions scattered all over the United States. One classmate applied to thirty-six surgical programs in twenty states. He was obsessed with "maximizing" his chances of admission to the most prestigious program possible. I remember asking how he had arrived at a rank order for all these places. His reply was understandably vague.

When he sends off his application form to residency programs, which oddly enough, ask little more than name, medical school, and social security number, the medical student has leaped into the "match." This experience is somewhat akin to Alice's strange fall through the rabbit hole. When the curious trip is over, you will be somewhere for sure, but as for just precisely where, well, that is anybody's guess. The match, a program by which virtually every hospital with a postgraduate training program abides, does not offer applicants the kind of flexibility they had in applying to college or medical school. Indeed, its very purpose is to eliminate the luxury of mulling over several letters of acceptance (and to minimize the chance that some hospitals will have too many interns and some not enough).

On the basis of their completed applications, including those "heavy" letters of recommendations, and even a few secretly placed phone calls between medical school professors, hospitals invite some applicants for an interview and write a polite brushoff to the rest. The amount of winnowing that takes place at this level varies tremendously. Some programs interview only a tiny percentage of all applicants; others agree to look over more than half.

The "interview trip" is a classic part of the autumn of the senior year. Some people buy fancy airline tickets and disappear for a month. Like barnstorming presidential candidates, they touch down in twenty cities in thirty days, pausing only for a weekend to test the powder at Aspen. For others it is a series of long drives each weekend to make Monday morning interviews in Rochester, Washington, Boston, and Baltimore. A few folks just can't seem to get into this scene. They take the train to New York City a couple of times and let matters rest.

Theoretically, the visit provides the student a chance to get a feel for the program. After an hour of the usual puffery of orientation, a quick tour of the facilities, and an interview or two with some bigshots, the student is free to ferret out whatever facts are available from the current interns, nurses, and medical students at that institution. The interns are by far the best source of information—if you allow for the fact that they are usually so depressed that no program sounds good.

In the middle of January comes a magic day by which the computers in Illinois demand to receive "rank-order" forms from all the medical students and all the training programs that have agreed to enter the match for that year. Despite the incredible amount of computer time it must take to run this program, the way the match algorithm works is simple. The students list, in order of their desire to train there, all the programs at which they interviewed. Similarly, the hospitals, in order of their desire to employ them, list the students that they would most like to have working as their interns. The lists are run against each other so that students are guaranteed a match with the hospital highest on their list that has not yet filled its intern quota. This is eminently fair, but it means that you had better think your preference list over with great care. It is the only way you have to control the outcome of the match. If you really don't want to train in a particular program, don't rank it, for you might wind up there.

There is one fact about the match that many senior medical students do not discover or, perhaps, refuse to believe: Many decent programs don't fill their intern quota. That is, after the computer has belched out its last match calculation, there are still some intern slots that many hospitals need to fill quickly. This means that it is foolish to list programs you really don't like just to increase the odds of matching. Rather than running the risk of getting a program you don't want, it is better not to match and enter the "free agent pool." Your bargaining power improves greatly. Just as when you were applying to college, you may pick and choose. Imagine what might happen if enough medical students actually played out their options in this fashion. As more students shortened their match lists, fewer programs would fill and the match program would lose its iron grip on the futures of 15,000 medical students. Programs would be forced to compete nakedly for interns! Perhaps salaries would go up and on-call duties would go down. Think about it—especially if you want to go to medical school!

A few weeks after the application and supporting letters have been sent out, the student learns which hospitals have decided to offer an interview. Of course, if the mailman brings a politely diplomatic brushoff, the future is a little less uncertain. The student will not be slaving at that particular hospital next year. If the letter is a sunny upbeat invitation to interview, the student, like the rookie at spring training, had made the first cut. When all the replies were in, it turned out that I had fared moderately well. Two Harvard programs had not offered me an interview. All the other programs on my short list (Dartmouth, Cornell, NYU, Yale, Boston University Hospital, Boston City Hospital, and the Mt. Auburn Hospital) were willing to take a closer look.

I began interviewing convinced that it would be nearly impossible to get any real "feel" for the various programs. I was wrong. After the visits were over I knew that of the seven residency programs, I was really only interested in two. I first visited Dartmouth, which trained people at the Mary Hitchcock Hospital in Hanover, New Hampshire, and the VA Hospital in White River Junction, Vermont. The hospital was beautiful, the professors were friendly, the ancillary services were excellent, and the nurses and house officers seemed to like the place. There were only two problems. While the patients, nearly all hardy, white Yankees, would be a pleasure to care for, the spectrum of illness that I would see there seemed less diverse than in a big city hospital. But that concern was less important to me than the matter of geography. Hanover, New Hampshire, is certainly one of the most beautiful places to live in the Northeast. But the town is tiny, the winter is long, and (even taking Dartmouth into account) the cultural diversions are limited. I knew that despite the town's Kodachrome loveliness, I would hunger for city lights.

From Hanover I made the long trek down the Connecticut River Valley to New York City. My first stop was the celebrated Bellevue Hospital, home of the New York University training program. Even though I had once lived in Manhattan for three years and had visited regularly during medical school, now that I was looking at them with the eyes of an intern, New York and Bellevue both seemed overwhelming. As I weaved my way through an endless stream of people who had come from every corner of the earth to crowd Second Avenue, and heard ambulance after ambulance scream past, a wave of anxiety broke over me. An hour later, during the standard hospital tour, the anxiety got a lot worse. The resident who was our host paused in the parking lot by the emergency room. He pointed to a big circle painted on the asphalt, saying, "That's where the helicopters land." Then he looked out at the East River and casually said, "that's where we get our drownings." The doors to the ER opened to another surprise. Instead of the wall of white coats I had expected, blue was the dominant color. There were at least twice as many cops as there were doctors. A rare and calming sense of certainty suffused me. I knew that I would not be training at NYU.

A week later, when I interviewed at the Cornell program, the city seemed a lot different. It was a quiet, sunny Saturday morning on the east side. New York Hospital towered in splendor over the surrounding residential neighborhood and the greens of Rockefeller University. The hospital reminded me vaguely of the great English cathedrals at Winchester and Canterbury. A pleasant receptionist ushered me along polished corridors to a sumptuous conference room. The table was laden with expensive pastries, and the coffee tasted unusually good. A bit later, one of the senior people in the Department of Medicine ushered me into his office and immediately began talking as though we were negotiating a seven-figure contract for the New York Yankees, an extremely flattering experience. I concluded that Cornell definitely had the sales pitch down to a science. The rest of the morning was equally impressive. The house officers were smooth, the ER was busy, but not too busy, and the wards were attractive. The visit to Sloan-Kettering, the world famous cancer center next door, was fascinating. Fantasies of being a great oncologist danced through my head. Cornell would be on my list.

The following week I visited three training programs in Boston. Mt. Auburn Hospital, a pleasant community hospital on the Charles River, a stone's throw from Harvard Square, was the only small program at which I was going to interview. It was staffed by superbly trained physicians, many of whom had simply opted for private practice in one of the nation's most stimulating communities rather than for the academic life. Here, too, the facilities were top notch, the doctors engaging, and the opportunities to learn more than adequate. Mt. Auburn also had the special attraction of a call schedule that required the intern in the house only every fourth night (a virtual vacation compared to every third night). Another big advantage of working there would be the opportunity to live in Cambridge, and to stroll occasionally past exquisite, old homes on tree-lined streets. If I could only shake the haunting pull of the "name" program that controls so many medical students, I might wind up there.

After Mt. Auburn Hospital I visited the two training programs associated with the Boston University School of Medicine. University Hospital is small, private, and research oriented; its people work in a comfortable, academic atmosphere that during my tour reminded me of Yale. But two things happened during my visit here that troubled me. Another medical student and I attended "morning report," the hour when the residents discuss management issues with an attending. For some reason neither the attending nor the residents bid us welcome or spoke to us after the session. This struck me as unfriendly. Later, when a senior resident gave us a quick tour of the hospital his praise of the program sounded hollow. When he explained to me that here interns admitted patients two out of three days, I began to lose interest.

Boston City Hospital, located only a hundred yards from University Hospital, was a completely different world. The hospital reminded me of a rusty old tramp steamer, still afloat after a hundred years. It was a warren of tired red brick buildings with a maze of endless corridors. Surely, it would take a year just to learn one's way around. The telltale signs of big city budget problems were everywhere. I entered a side door with a broken window, the corridor walls had not seen fresh paint since the Korean War, and I found the secretary of the physician with whom my interview had been scheduled wrapped in her winter coat. A boiler was broken, and the offices in that building had not felt heat in three weeks. Throughout the hospital the message was repeated: Money was extremely tight. I cringed.

Oddly enough, the interns seemed unperturbed by the desperate physical circumstances under which they worked. There was a real team spirit in the air. Or was I just talking with pathological optimists? Because I knew two former Yale students who were working here, I had a special line on reality. I found Ernie working in the cramped ICU. As he searched futilely for a vein in the arm of a patient with hepatic encephalopathy, he offered me his assessment.

"No matter where you go, internship shits. There is no way around it. I was disappointed when I matched here, but I've grown to love the place. The house staff is great, the attendings are not condescending, and you get a lot of responsibility fast. Plus, the night float [a system in which each intern spends three weeks of the year working a twelve-hour night shift that relieves the on-call intern of his or her admitting responsibilities and promises at least a couple of hours of sleep] really protects you."

Bert, my other friend, confirmed Ernie's opinion.

What really sold me on Boston City Hospital was my

interview. The doctor was a young British cardiologist with a wispy blond beard and a warm smile. We hit it off at once. For the next hour we had one of those rare conversations in which two strangers seem to be mind-readers. The interview spilled way over its allotted time and ended only when I was called to another meeting. A veteran of several training programs, including the famous Peter Bent Brigham Hospital, he convinced me that Boston City was the best place he knew to learn the basics of internal medicine.

By mid-December the interview season was over. I was back in New Haven spending endless hours trying to recall and reassess my first impressions of the various programs and filling page after page with tentative preference lists. Throughout the autumn I had steadfastly refused to apply to Yale. I believed that it would be better to get my postgraduate training at a new institution. There are, after all, few opportunities to get a fresh start in life. But at the last minute I crumbled. As I remembered the budget problems at Boston City Hospital, the isolation of Hanover, and the kaleidoscopic style of Manhattan, Yale seemed friendly and reliable. The thought of being an intern in a strange hospital was very frightening.

On the last possible day I had my Yale interview. Few experiences are so thoroughly predictable. Year after year the same professor interviews all the applicants to Yale's residency in medicine who are Yale students. Over the years he has perfected a ten-minute discussion of "your chances of training here," which has acquired folk-tale status among fourth-year students. An hour or so before the interview, my friend Rob told me what I would hear.

"There are basically three groups of Yale students. There are two or three who have fooled everybody for four years.

They are going to be accepted. There are a few more who have fooled nobody in four years. They don't have a chance. Then there is everyone else: the people who have solid but imperfect credentials. They will have a chance to get in, but it is impossible to predict who will win the lottery. I estimate that you are in the middle of the middle group."

How helpful, I thought.

I waited about ten minutes before being ushered into the tiny cluttered office of one of the world's leading clinical researchers. He lost no time letting me know that I was the twenty-eighth Yale senior he had spoken to, and he was tired of it. His blunt demeanor was perfectly understandable. After all, if Yale students were eager to continue training in New Haven, why waste energy being diplomatic? I politely listened to the spiel, which closely tracked Rob's descriptions, thanked my professor and left. The interview had had a beneficial effect. My resolve to move on had returned.

A few weeks later, after countless hours of rumination and list manipulation, I finally sat down to fill out the damn match form so it would be postmarked on time to satisfy the computers. The rules said you had to list every program in which you had interviewed. However, by placing an X in an appropriate spot you could eliminate any program from consideration. After mailing in this list, there was one last opportunity to delete programs, but no other changes were permitted.

In the late night winter stillness of my apartment, the task seemed impossible. The more I thought about them, the more the imponderables of unknown programs frightened me. Again, I forgot my resolve. New Haven had been my home for years. Life here was an easy compromise between big city and country. Despite my criticisms, the medical training program was superb. I decided to retain my chance of staying in New Haven. I marked Yale first and commenced a struggle with myself about how to list the others. When the emotional dust settled, I had ranked Boston City Hospital next, followed by Cornell, Boston University Hospital, Mt. Auburn Hospital, and Dartmouth. Last came NYU, next to which I put an X. I quickly sealed the envelope and walked briskly to the corner mailbox. It was done.

A peaceful empty feeling settled in immediately. The matter was out of my hands. Miraculously, I was again able to think of other subjects. The newspaper became interesting. I found pleasure in the crisp air and distant January sun. For several weeks life seemed normal. Neither I nor my classmates could hear the computer whirring in its aseptic, concrete home in an Illinois cornfield. As ordained, one day the peace shattered. The postal service, for once too accurate, delivered a computerized restatement of our match forms back to us. My future was before me. There was only one question to decide: Did I wish to delete any programs?

The deadline for the *final* return of the match form came in late February as I was floundering through my subinternship. One of our professors had advised a fellow student, "Never do your sub when you are trying to decide on the match because you will be too heavily influenced by the trauma of your first clinical responsibilities." She was right. The sub had helped to quench my desire to stay at Yale. Although I knew it would probably be no rougher to train here than elsewhere, I wanted out. Again on the last night that I could possibly delay before posting my list, I deleted Yale and Dartmouth. I was now down to only four programs, a very short match list. The decision to eliminate Dartmouth hardly mattered. But by ending all chance of going to Yale, I had chosen my own fate. The die had been cast when I ranked Boston City Hospital ahead of

Cornell. Unless there were a nuclear war, I felt certain that I would be an intern at Boston City Hospital the following July.

Match day fell on March 18. At the time I was two thousand miles away from the mailroom in Yale Medical School, where the match results were distributed. My friend, Dick, whom I had asked to open my envelope, called me with the news: It was Boston City Hospital.

Match day is a day of triumph and defeat. Most students match. But, for the first time in their lives some medical students do not clear an academic hurdle. It is a day when many people swell with pride. A few others try hard to wear the mask of happiness, however loosely it fits. For everyone there is also a sudden rushing wind of change. Warm waves of nostalgia wash over us. Incredible! Medical school is over. A new world beckons.

...*In all dangerous cases you should be on the watch for all favourable coctions of the evacuations from all parts, or for fair and critical abscessions. Coctions signify nearness of crisis and sure recovery of health, but crude and unconcocted evacuations, which change into bad abscessions, denote absence of crisis, pain, prolonged illness, death, or a return of the same symptoms. But it is by a consideration of other signs that one must decide which of these results will be most likely. Declare the past, diagnose the present, foretell the future; practise these acts. As to diseases, make a habit of two things—to help, or at least* to do no harm. *The art has three factors, the disease, the patient, the physician. The physician is the servant of the art. The patient must co-operate with the physician in combating the disease.*

From *Hippocrates,*
"Epidemics I," translated
by W. H. S. Jones in the
Loeb Classical Library
(Cambridge: Harvard
University Press, 1923).

*I swear by Apollo Physician, by Asclepius, by Health,
by Panacea and by all the gods and goddesses, making
them my witnesses, that I will carry out, according to
my ability and judgment, this oath and this indenture.
To hold my teacher in this art equal to my own
parents; to make him partner in my livelihood; when
he is need of money to share mine with him; to
consider his family as my own brothers, and to teach
them this art, if they want to learn it, without fee or
indenture; to impart precept, oral instruction, and all
other instruction to my own sons, the sons of my
teacher, and to indentured pupils who have taken the
physician's oath, but to nobody else. I will use
treatment to help the sick according to my ability and
judgment, but never with a view to injury and wrong-
doing. Neither will I administer a poison to anybody
when asked to do so, nor will I suggest such a course.
Similarly I not give to a woman a pessary to cause
abortion. But I will keep pure and holy both my life
and my art. I will not use the knife, not even, verily, on
sufferers from stone, but I will give place to such as are
craftsmen therein. Into whatsoever houses I enter, I
will enter to help the sick, and I will abstain from all
intentional wrong-doing and harm, especially from
abusing the bodies of man or woman, bond or free.
And whatsoever I shall see or hear in the course of my
profession, as well as outside my profession in my
intercourse with men, if it be what should not be
published abroad, I will never divulge, holding such
things to be holy secrets. Now if I carry out this oath,
and break it not, may I gain for ever reputation among
all men for my life and for my art; but if I transgress it
and foreswear myself, may the opposite befall me.*

From *Hippocrates,* "Oath,"
translated by W. H. S. Jones in the
Loeb Classical Library (Cambridge:
Harvard University Press, 1923).